Handbook of Practical Biochemistry

Handbook of Practical Biochemistry

Deepti Saini
Department of Biochemistry
All India Institute of Medical Sciences
New Delhi

Deepak K Saini
PhD
Department of Biotechnology
All India Institute of Medical Sciences
New Delhi

PEEPEE
PUBLISHERS and DISTRIBUTORS (P) LTD.

Handbook Practical Biochemistry

Published by
Pawaninder P. Vij

Peepee Publishers and Distributors (P) Ltd.
Head Office: 160, Shakti Vihar, Pitam Pura
Delhi - 110 034 (India)

Correspondence Address:

7/31, First Floor
Ansari Road, Daryaganj, Post Box-7243
New Delhi-110 002 (India)

Ph: 65195868, 23246245, 9811156083

e-mail: peepee160@yahoo.co.in

e-mail: peepee160@rediffmail.com

e-mail: peepee160@gmail.com

www.peepeepub.com

First Edition: 2004
Reprint: **2009**

ISBN: 81-88867-15-2

Printed at
Lordson, C-5/19, Rana Pratap Bagh, Delhi-110007

PREFACE

With the advent of new technologies, more and more reliable diagnostic techniques and tools are now available to the clinicians. As of today there is no physician who relies merely on his/her medical instincts to diagnose his/her patients. Thanks to the advancements in the science of medicine laboratory diagnosis has gained tremendous importance in today's clinical practice. It does not need a specialist today to link the disease processes to biochemical changes in the body fluids. It is now considered of utmost importance for all physicians to have a detailed biochemical investigation performed on his/her patients before ascertaining the disease condition.

In this context, we are hopeful that this short book covering various aspects of practical biochemistry would come handy to all medical biochemistry students, practicing physicians and clinical biochemists as well. We have also tried to arrange the book as a handy manual with a simple self guided approach to various aspects of practical biochemistry.

We are grateful to the generous help provided by various individuals from our field, who have helped in bringing this book in the current form.

Deepti Saini
Deepak K Saini

Metabolic changes associated with specific disorders may give rise to a change in the biochemical profile of a particular body fluid, e.g. elevated blood glucose in diabetes mellitus or reduced glucose levels in the cerebrospinal fluid in bacterial meningitis. Hence, specific parameters are looked for in a specific body fluid when a disease is suspected. Nowadays, physicians generally refer a patient for a battery of biochemical investigations which could reveal predisposition to specific disease processes, e.g. elevated levels of SGOT/ SGPT for a long time can indicate towards the development of liver disorder.

From a clinical point of view, one purpose of performing a test could be corroborating a particular diagnosis or ruling it out. Other tests may be done to assess the severity of a disease process or monitor its progress. Still others may evaluate or monitor the effectiveness or potential side effects of a particular therapeutic regimen; and certain tests can give a clue about the prognosis or probable outcome of a disease.

In a standard clinical biochemistry lab, there should be certain standard operating procedures (SOP) which should be followed irrespective of the person performing the assay or the test. SOP is a clear, concise and comprehensive written instruction of a method or procedure which has been agreed upon and authorized as the operating policy of the department. In general, SOPs, which mainly contain detailed descriptions of each analytical method, are essential for maintaining the same analytical quality over a long period of time. A standard set of procedure can include the following parameters:

- Technique and its principle
- Nature and type of sample which can be used in the assay including its storage and preservation
- Requirements, preparation of reagents, their storage and stability
- Specialized equipment required for the analysis and their functioning
- Detailed protocol
- A calibration curve for the assay and analytical reliability
- Standard values (reference range and its clinical significance)
- Interfering agents for the assay and their effect on the outcome of result.

With these conditions laid out clearly before start of every assay there is not reason to doubt your experimentation under any circumstances, because as a biochemist you need to be absolutely certain about finding, as even an iota of unreliability might affect the clinical findings of the disease and can consequently jeopardize the patient's well being.

CONTENTS

Part—I:

Introduction to Clinical Biochemistry

1

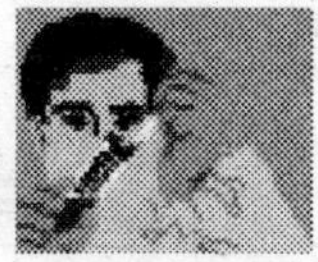

Specimen Collection, Handling, Storage and Processing

Since many factors might affect the outcome of clinical analysis of body fluids, it is of utmost importance to the biochemist to take precautions and follow certain set guidelines used for collection, storing and processing samples for biochemical evaluation. For example, if the blood collected is to be used for estimation of serum insulin levels, then it should be stored at 4°C or lower and not at room temperature as routinely followed.

Following is a broad tabulation of types of samples, investigations which can be performed with them, their mode of collection and storage. The detail in the Table 1.1 does not limit the types of samples or tests which can be performed with them.

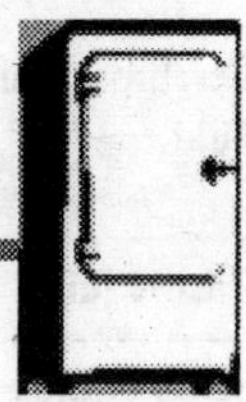

PRESERVATION OF SAMPLES: GENERAL PRINCIPLE

Alteration in the concentration or activity of a constituent in a stored specimen can result from various natural processes such as:

1. Adsorption on to the glass container.
2. Evaporation if the constituent is volatile such as O_2 and CO. This can be prevented or at least slowed by collection and storage of samples under anaerobic conditions.
3. Water shift due to the addition of anticoagulants.
4. Metabolic activities of the erythrocytes and leukocytes (accelerated by hemolysis) inducing O_2 consumption and CO production, hydrolysis, glycolysis and finally degradation.
5. Microbial (fungal/bacterial) growth–This appears when the sample is to be stored for longer than one day either at room or refrigerator

Table 1.1: Listing of types of samples, investigation types and the method/s of collection and storage of sample.

Body fluid	*Investigations*	*Method of collection and storage*
Whole blood	Blood gases Glucose Urea	Obtained by arterial or venepuncture; collected with anticoagulants like heparin, etc.
	Genetic abnormalities	Store at 4°C or -20°C for long term.
Plasma	Enzymes Metabolites Electrolyte	Blood is collected with anticoagulants, centrifuged at 2000 rpm and the supernatant fraction collected is plasma.
Serum	Enzymes Metabolites Electrolyte	Blood collected in plain glass container, without any anticoagulant, centrifuged at 2000 rpm after clotting, the serum 'supernatant' is collected.
Urine	Sugar Proteins Bile salts Pigments Blood steroids	Directly passed into a glass container or sometimes a catheter is introduced in the bladder. Storage at 4°C.
Cerebrospinal fluid	Sugar Protein Chloride	Lumbar puncture.
Gastric juice	HCl	Aspiration by Ryle's tube, blood
Serous fluids	Proteins	Needle puncture to the serous space. (e.g. pleural, peritoneal)
Sweat	Chloride	Soaked into a filter paper
Amniotic fluid	Genetic abnormalities	Ultrasonographically guided needle aspirate; 4°C or –20°C

temperature. This can be solved by following alternative courses of action, such as:

a. Collection and storage under sterile conditions,
b. Freezing of the sample,
c. Extreme alteration of pH and
d. Addition of an antibacterial agent.

In extreme cases samples can be lyophilized, such samples are stable with respect to many constituents for periods of at least ten years. Though degradation at low temperature is considerably less (at refrigerator temperature) and is completely inhibited in the frozen state, but even in the frozen state, some components of plasma deteriorate. Besides these physical preservation processes, chemical preservatives can also be used to prevent bacterial growth in samples. In 1923, Sanders introduced the combination of 10 mg sodium fluoride + 1 mg thymol/ml of blood as preservative. The presence of thymol effectively controlled microbial growth so that non-sterile specimens were stable for all determinations (except non-protein nitrogen) for at least two weeks. Monochlorobenzene and monobromobenzene have also been coupled with fluoride and have been claimed to be superior to thymol. Besides these, antibiotics like 1 mg of streptomycin base/ 10 ml of blood has been used for preservation of blood for hemoglobin and urea determinations. For urine specimens, the common preservatives used are formaldehyde, thymol, toluene and chloroform which primarily act as antimicrobial agents.

Preservation and Storage of Blood

Use of Anticoagulants

Chemical agents that prevent coagulation are routinely used when whole blood or plasma is required. Some of the commonly used anticoagulants are (i) Heparin (ii) salts of ethylene diamine tetra-acetic acid (EDTA), (iii) Oxalates and (iv) Sodium fluoride, (v) Sodium citrate and (vi) Sodium iodoacetate.

i. *Heparin.* It may be considered to be a natural anticoagulant because it is already present in the blood, but in concentrations less than that required to prevent clotting in freshly drawn blood. Heparin prevents coagulation by increasing the activity of antithrombin III, an inhibitor of thrombin. This anticoagulant is used in a concentration of 0.2 mg/ml of blood. If the blood has to be used for PCR diagnostics of various genetic abnormalities then it is not the anticoagulant of choice because heparin is a known inhibitor of PCR reaction and even trace amounts of heparin can inhibit the reaction.

ii. *Salts of ethylene diamine tetra-acetic acid (EDTA).* It is an anticoagulant which acts by virtue of removing calcium ions, an essential component of the clotting process, through chelation. A concentration of 2 mg of the disodium salt/ml of blood is sufficient for its anticoagulative activity. Concentrations even greater than this produce no detectable change in erythrocyte volume and shown no effect on the cellular components of blood.

iii. *Oxalates.* Lithium, sodium and potassium oxalates act as anticoagulants by removing calcium ions essential for blood coagulation. Potassium oxalate is the most commonly used salt and ~ 1-2 mg of salt/ml of blood is required. The disadvantage of the use of oxalate is the alteration of concentrations of plasma components. Shrinkage of erythrocytes results from a water shift from the erythrocytes to plasma. This shift increases with increasing anticoagulant concentration, and if used in the same concentration on a weight basis, all anticoagulants will have this effect inversely proportional to their molecular weight. Aside from the water shift there may be alteration of erythrocyte permeability, which may explain the varied and inconsistent effects of oxalates and other salt anticoagulants on certain plasma constituents. Besides these oxalate salts can also inhibit the activity of several enzymes including alkaline and acid phosphatases, amylase and lactate dehydrogenase.

iv. *Sodium fluoride.* It is used when blood is collected for glucose estimations as it inhibits the enzymes involved in glycolysis. In the erythrocytes (RBCs), it specifically inhibits the enzyme enolase of the glycolytic pathway, preventing the consumption of glucose by the RBCs. If blood is left standing at room temperature, the blood glucose level can decrease at a maximal rate 10 mg/dl/hr in absence of an antiglycolytic agent. This rate can be still higher in case of blood collected from newborns and leukemia patients due to the higher metabolic rates of their erythrocytes. Though it has a weak anticoagulant action, it is usually combined with another anticoagulant such as potassium oxalate.

v. *Sodium citrate.* It is used widely as its effect is reversible by addition of Ca^{2+} ions.

vi. *Sodium iodoacetate.* When glucose and urea has to be estimated from a single sample then sodium iodoacetate is used at a concentration of 2 mg/ml of blood as it is an effective antiglycolytic agent and has no effect on urease, whose activity is altered by sodium fluoride.

Effect of Hemolysis

Lysis of erythrocytes leading of liberation of free hemoglobin in serum in concentrations excess of 20 mg/ml is considered as hemolytic serum. Though at lower levels of hemolysis test values of most of the tests are not affected but in conditions of severe hemolysis certain test values might be altered. For the constituents whose concentration is less in the RBCs, the hemolysis brings about a reduction in their values because of a dilution effect and the converse the true for the constituents whose concentrations are high within the RBCs. Thus, the final concentrations of enzymes like lactate dehydrogenase, aldolase, acid phosphatases and electrolytes like Mg^{2+} and Ca^{2+} are particularly affected by hemolysis.

In the isolation of DNA for PCR diagnostics, hemolysis has severe effect since hemoglobin is an inhibitor of the PCR reaction by virtue of the interaction of Fe and pyrrole rings (present in hemoglobin) with Taq polymerase. Due to these undesired effects of hemolysis care should be taken so that minimum lysis of RBCs is caused.

Storage of Blood or its Fractions

Plasma and serum should be separated from the cells as soon as possible and stored at 4°C until analyzed. Though activity of some of the enzymes might be more stable at room temperature.

Preservation and Storage of Urine

Collection of urine sample depends on the nature of test desired. For microscopic examination and elucidation of presence of abnormally high amounts of protein, etc. a concentrated sample is desired. Such a sample can be obtained in early morning from the fasting patient as it is the most concentrated specimen.

Urine can be stored by simple refrigeration at 4°C, if the sample is to be processed the same day. Otherwise, depending about the nature of test, different types of preservatives can be used. For Ca^{2+} and steroid analysis and level determination, samples can be stored by acidification to pH below 3, whereas sodium bicarbonate can be used to preserve porphyrins and urobilinogen.

Preservation and Storage of Solid Tissues and/or Other Bodily Fluids

Solid tissues from many body parts are generally obtained by means of biopsies to study various malignancies. Such tissues should be stored immediately on ice after collection and should be frozen in liquid nitrogen within 20 minutes.

Spinal, synovial, amniotic, pleural, pericardial or ascitic fluids should be collected and stored on ice as soon as possible. These fluids are generally collected for investigating various immunological disorders like arthritis, inflammatory disorders, and presence of infectious agents or for congenital disorders. For all these analyses the samples can be safely stored at 4°C for short duration and -20°C for long periods.

2

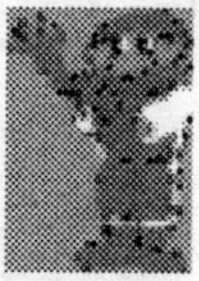

Safety Issues and Precautions for Clinical Biochemistry

Safety is an important issue even in a small clinical laboratory and it is advised that every clinical laboratory must have a formal safety program and it should be ensured that laboratory environment meets the accepted safety standards and the equipments in use are procured only from established manufacturers. Besides these, other details should also be addressed; such as:

1. Labeling and storage temperature of chemicals
2. Types and location of fire extinguishers
3. Condition of sterile containment hoods
4. Proper working and grounding of electrical equipment
5. Means and process for proper handling and disposal of bio-hazardous materials including specimen collected from patients and biowaste.

Besides these prechecks there are a number of other safety measures which should be taken to avoid/prevent chemical, electrical and biological hazards.

Chemicals

- Under no circumstances any chemical should be touched with bare hands or inhaled directly.
- Chemicals which are hazardous should be clearly marked in terms of nature of danger, e.g. do not inhale or do not expose to light.
- Proper storage of chemicals should be followed to prevent loss of their activity.
- Knowledge of the properties of chemicals in use and of proper handling procedures greatly reduces dangerous situations, e.g. preparation of a dilute solution of sulfuric acid needs the knowledge that water cannot be added to sulfuric acid for dilution as it would lead to spontaneous explosion, rather it should be diluted by adding

acid slowly into water with stirring to avoid explosion and consequential burns.

- All the corrosive and hazardous chemicals should be stored separately within the provided containment containers.
- Do not try to solubilize any chemical in a solvent unless the solubility properties are known and do not heat the solution to enhance the solubility unless otherwise recommended, e.g. 40% acrylamide might take time to dissolve but never heat the solution to enhance solubility as acrylamide explodes on heating.

Electrical

- All the electrical equipments should be grounded using three-point plugs and use of the extension cord should be avoided.
- Use the equipment at the recommended voltage only; do not exceed the recommended voltage.
- Do not install heat generating electrical equipments such as centrifuges and power packs, etc. in closed places. There should be proper air circulation around the equipment to minimize the heating.
- Do not operate any electrical appliance with wet hands; it may lead to electrical shock.
- Operate all sensitive equipments with power back up systems to protect them from damage in case of power failure.

Biological

Biological hazards can be avoided by following 'universal precautions'.

- All specimens should be treated as potentially infectious and hazardous.
- Never perform mouth pipetting or blow out pipettes that contain potentially infectious material, e.g. serum.
- Do not mix potentially infectious material by bubbling air through the liquid, which leads to aerosol formation.
- Barrier protection such as gloves, mask, protective eyewear and gowns must be used when taking any sample from a patient. Disposable, nonsterile latex or vinyl gloves, facemask and a protective gown provide adequate protection.
- Wash hands whenever gloves are changed and disposed.
- Facial barrier protection should be used if there is a significant potential for the spattering of the blood or body fluid.

- Avoid using syringes whenever possible and dispose off needles in rigid containers without touching.
- Dispose off all sharp objects appropriately.
- Make a habit of keeping your hands away from your mouth, nose, eye and any other mucous membranes. This will reduce the possibility of infection.
- Decontaminate all surfaces and reusable devices after use with appropriate registered hospital disinfectant.
- No warning labels are to be used on patient specimens, but all of them should be treated as potentially hazardous.
- Before centrifuging, inspect tubes for cracks, the inside of caps for signs of erosion or adhering matter and the rubber cushions for any deposits, which might lead to sample contamination or sample loss.
- Never leave a discarded tube or infected material unattended or unlabeled.
- Periodically clean out freezer and dry ice chests to remove broken ampules and tubes of biological samples. Use rubber gloves and respiratory protection during this cleaning.

Other Precautions

Every laboratory should have the necessary equipments to put out a fire in the laboratory, as well as to put out a fire on the clothing of an individual. Easy access to extinguishers should be made and if possible a specific person should be assigned the job of laboratory safety officer.

3

Data Collection and Presentation

Presentation of Results

Data presentation should be crisp and should include the standard values for immediate reference. The results should be presented in an internationally accepted format given under.

1. Metabolites (glucose, urea, etc.) are expressed as mg/dL or mmol/L.
2. Electrolytes (Na^+/K^+) as mmol/L.
3. Enzymes as units/L [Enzymes are sometimes expressed in conventional units (e.g. Amylase in Somogy units, phosphatase in King-Armstrong units)].

Interpretation of Results

Values obtained with a particular parameter are interpreted as increased, decreased or within normal (reference) range. Reference values are obtained from individuals who are in good health as judged by other clinical and laboratory parameters, after suitable standardization and statistical analysis, under definite laboratory conditions. These values are now quite well defined for all the tests routinely performed in clinical biochemistry labs. Normal (Reference) range is the value within which 95% normal healthy persons fall. Physiological factors like age and gender, exercise, posture, circadian variations, food, drugs and stimulants and effect of underlying medical conditions may effect the interpretation of results.

Quality Control

A major role of the clinical laboratory is the measurement of substances in body fluids or tissues for the purpose of diagnosis, treatment or prevention of disease, and for greater understanding of the disease process. To fulfill these aims the data generated has to be reliable for which strict quality control has to be maintained. Quality control is defined briefly as the control of those sources of variation, which are the responsibility of the laboratory, and the procedures used to recognize and minimize them.

Accuracy. It is the degree of agreement between a measured value and its 'true/consensus' value. On the contrary, inaccuracy, which is represented by analytical bias, is defined as the percentage of the difference between the measured value and the 'true' value over the true value. Therefore, good accuracy means less analytical error.

Precision. It refers to reproducibility. It refers to the agreement between replicate measurements. It is quantitatively expressed as the standard deviation (SD) or more precisely as percent coefficient of variation (CV), which is defined as SD times 100 divided by the mean value of the results in a set of replicate measurements. Therefore, good precision means least CV.

Accuracy has to do with how close the mean of a sufficiently large number of determinations on a sample is to be the actual amount of substance present and is dependent on the methodology used. Precision refers to the extent to which repeated determination on an individual specimen vary using a particular technique and is dependent on how rigorously the methodology is followed.

Sensitivity and Specificity

No test is completely accurate all of the time. Sometimes a test result indicates an abnormal value in a person who does not have the suspected disease, which indicates towards a 'false-positive' result. Sometimes a test result indicates a normal value in a person who has the disease, i.e. a 'false-negative' result. Tests are rated in terms of their *sensitivity* which is the probability that their results will be positive when a disease is present and their *specificity*, the probability that their results will be negative when a disease is not present. A very sensitive test is unlikely to miss the disease in people who have it, however, it may falsely indicate disease in healthy people. A very specific test is unlikely to indicate disease in healthy people. Although, it may miss the disease in some who have it. Problems with sensitivity and specificity can be largely overcome by using several different tests.

Because your physician cannot always be sure whether or not the reported result of a particular test from a particular person is false or true, a person with an abnormal result may often need to be re-tested or undergo a different type of testing.

Normal test result values are generally expressed as a reference range, which is based on the average values in a healthy population and 95% of healthy people have values within this range. These values might vary somewhat among laboratories, due to methodology and even geography. Tests and testing vary widely in different parts of the world, and in different parts of most countries, due to characteristics in the population, among other factors.

Part—II:
Instrumentation and Techniques

4

pH Measurement and Buffer Solutions

The maintenance of a stable hydrogen ion concentration in the body fluids is essential for life. The pH of a solution is the value which defines this hydrogen ion concentration. In an aqueous solution, it is the relative 'strengths' of the hydrogen ion rich species called 'acid' and the hydrogen ion deficient species called 'base' which determines the net pH of a solution.

Acids and bases are proton donor and proton acceptor species respectively.

Each acid has a conjugate base, i.e. Acid = Base + H^+

Alkali yields hydroxyl ions on dissociation. $KOH \rightarrow K^+ + OH^-$

Ampholytes is ionic species that can act both as acids and bases.

Strong acid or stròng base completely ionize in solution, so that concentration of free H^+ or OH^- is the same as the concentration of the acid or base. e.g. HNO_3, NaOH.

Weak acid or weak base dissociate to a limited extent and the concentration of free H^+ or OH^- depends on the dissociation constant, e.g. HCOOH, $C_6H_6NH_2$.

Biological systems involve aqueous media hence, in most biochemical calculations, the strength of an acid is in reference to water as a solvent.

pH. The negative logarithm of the hydrogen ion activity, but in practice hydrogen ion concentration is usually taken. If $H^+ = 0.398 \times 10^{-7}$, then pH =-log $(0.398 \times 10^{-7}) = 7.4$

In aqueous solutions pH ranges from 0 to 14.

K_w (dissociation constant of water). At 25°C water is very weakly ionized and H^+ is only 10^{-7} mol/ L. The equilibrium constant for this dissociation:

$K = \frac{[H^+][OH^-]}{[H_2O]}$ or $K_w = [H^+][OH^-]$, since concentration of water is constant.

Temperature and K_w. Ionic product of pure water at 25°C is 10^{-14}, so that pH is 7. At other temperatures pH at neutrality is not 7 since K_w varies with temperature. A temperature change from 37° to 40°C causes 8% rise in H^+ and OH^-. Hence a slight rise or fall in temperature may cause a profound biological change in a system sensitive to H^+.

Dissociation constant of a weak acid The relative strength of an acid is expressed as dissociation constant. For a weak acid HA, dissociation constant

$$K = \frac{[H^+][A^-]}{[HA]},$$

and is expressed as pK=–log K.

Lower the pK, stronger is the acid.

Relationship of pH to pK. The Henderson-Hasselbalch equation gives a relation ship

$$pH = pK + \log \frac{[salt]}{[acid]}$$

Derivation:

$K = \frac{[H^+][A^-]}{[HA]}$ where HA is a weak acid and dissociates into H^+ & A^-

or

$$[H^+] = K \frac{[HA]}{[A^-]}$$

or

$$-\log [H^+] = -\log K \frac{[HA]}{[A^-]}$$

or

$$pH = -\log K - \log \frac{[HA]}{[A^-]}$$

or

$$pH = pK - \log \frac{[HA]}{[A^-]} \text{ or } pH = pK + \log \frac{[A^-]}{[HA]}$$

Application. To calculate pH, pK or molar ratio of H^+ donor and acceptor.

Measurement of pH

pH Indicators

pH indicators are usually organic compounds of natural or synthetic origin whose color is dependent on the pH of the solution. Indicators are usually weak acids which dissociate in solution.

Indicator = $\text{Indicator}^- + H^+$ and $pH = pK_{In} + \log \frac{[\text{Indicator}^-]}{[\text{Indicator}]}$, with both forms of the indicator having different color. The actual color of the solution will depend on the pK_{In} and the pH. Indicators are most useful around the pK_{In}. Disadvantages of indicators are that they are approximate indications of pH, since color change takes place over a wide pH range and that they are affected by oxidizing agents, reducing agents, salts and proteins. Indicators should be used in small quantities, so that the acid-base equilibrium of the test solution is not displaced. Hence, indicators are best used in determining end point of titrations. e.g. BPB (Bromo phenol blue) is yellow colored in acidic pH and blue at alkaline pH.

pH Meter

The most reliable and accurate method for the routine measurement of pH is the pH meter in which a change in pH is measured as a change in electrical potential.

If a metal rod is placed in a solution of its salts, it acquires potential. If two dissimilar metals are dipped into the solutions of their salts, the difference in potential can be measured or calculated from the two separate potentials. A standard electrode is thus required against which the potential of all other electrodes can be compared. This is the standard hydrogen electrode, consisting of a platinum rod dipped in an aqueous solution with a given H^+ activity in which Hydrogen gas is bubbled continuously at 1 atmosphere pressure. But as this is too cumbersome to be used as a reference electrode for routine use, other secondary reference electrodes of known potential in relation to the standard hydrogen electrodes are used.

Calomel electrode. The most commonly used secondary reference electrode is the calomel electrode consisting of mercury-mercurous chloride in contact with a saturated solution of KCl. Its potential is pH independent.

Glass electrode. In the pH meter, the most commonly used pH dependent unit is the glass electrode. It consists of a very thin bulb about 0.1 mm thick blown on to a glass tube of high resistance. Inside the bulb is a solution of HCl (0.1 M) connected to a platinum wire via a silver-silver chloride electrode, which is reversible to H^+. The electrode is made from certain types of borosilicate glass permeable to H^+ but not to other cations and anions. Therefore, if a thin glass membrane separates two solutions of different pH, a potential difference is generated across the membrane the magnitude of which is given by the equation.

$$E = 2.303 \frac{RT}{F} \log \frac{[H^+]_i}{[H^+]_o}$$

Where E = potential, R = gas constant, T = absolute temperature F = Faraday constant $[H^+]_i$= concentration on the inside which is fixed (O.1N HCl), and $[H^+]_o$ = concentration on the outside (test sample).

The voltage measured by such a system is primarily the difference between that of the glass and, the reference electrodes (other fixed potentials in the circuit also contribute) and it is linearly related to the pH of the test solution, i.e. $[H^+]_o$. The system therefore consists of the glass electrode in contact with the solution to be measured, the calomel reference electrode, a KCl bridge (the KCl should flow slowly into the sample) and the measuring device (meter). These are designed so that pH 7 gives a zero potential. High resistances (10^6-10^8 Omega) are used so that very little current is drawn from the circuit. (A large current flow could change the ion concentration).

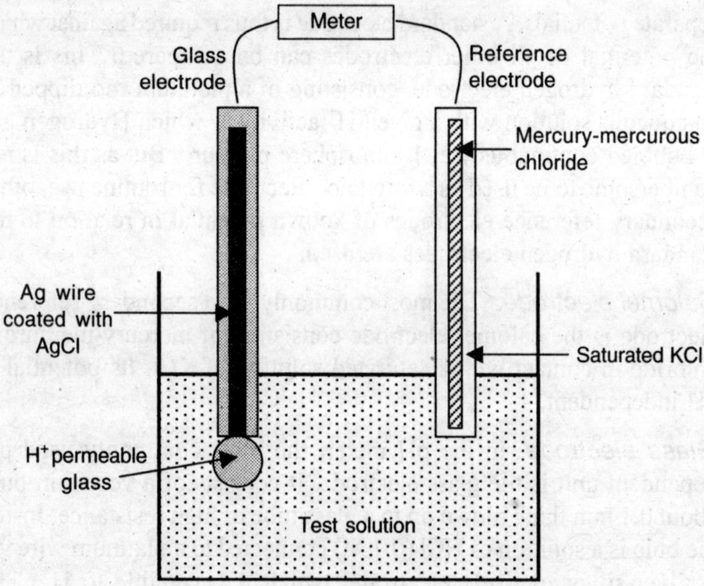

Fig. 4.1: General configuration of a pH meter

Precautions

Certain precautions have to be observed while using a pH meter. The glass electrode is fragile and must be handled with care. New electrodes must be soaked in 0.1 M HCl several hours before use. Electrodes must not be left to dry. Glass electrode is usually kept dipped in 3M KCl. The temperature compensation dial must be set before it is calibrated as potential produced is dependent on temperature. The meter must be calibrated first with a standard buffer pH 7, and then with a standard of pH 4 (if the test sample is expected to be acidic) or with a standard of pH 9 or 10 (if test is expected to be basic). Electrodes must be washed with distilled water before and after use. For storage, the pH meter should be switched to zero but the main switch left on.

Buffer Solutions

Buffers are defined as substances that resist changes in the pH of the system. Weak acids or bases, in the presence of their salts with strong base or strong acid respectively form buffer systems. For example, phosphate/monohydrogen phosphate, carbonic acid/bicarbonate, proteins/proteinate.

The action of buffers and their role in maintaining the pH of a solution can best be explained with the aid of the Henderson-Hasselbalch equation:

$$pH = pK + \log \frac{[A^-]}{[HA]} \quad \text{or} \quad pH = pK + \log \frac{[\text{salt}]}{[\text{acid}]}$$

where [salt] = $[A^-]$ = concentration of dissociated salt and [acid] = [HA] = concentration of undissociated acid.

The pH of the system is determined by the pK of the acid and the ratio of $[A^-]$ to [HA]. The buffer has greatest buffering capacity at its pK, the pH at which the $[A^-]$ = [HA]

$$pH = pK + \log 1$$

The capacity of the buffer decreases as the ratio deviates from 1. In general, buffers should be used at a pH ± 1 from the pK. If the ratio is beyond 50:1 or 1:50, the system is considered to have lost its buffering capacity.

Common Laboratory Buffers

The pH in many biological experiments often needs to be kept constant in the range of pH 6-8, but there are few weak acids or bases that are effective buffers at this part of the pH scale, particularly around pH 7.4, the pH of blood.

1. *Bicarbonate* buffer spontaneously liberates CO_2 and should be maintained in an atmosphere of CO_2. pK_a is 6.1, so the buffering capacity around pH 7.4 is poor.
2. *Phosphate* buffer is probably the most popular buffer but phosphate readily forms complexes with heavy metals. It can act as an activator, inhibitor of metabolite of many biochemical reactions. Buffering capacity is poor above pH 7.5.
3. *Tris* buffer can be used with heavy metals, but can act as inhibitor in some biochemical systems. Tris has high lipid solubility and penetrates membranes. Temperature effect is the major disadvantage. Tris buffer pH 7.8 at RT has a pH of 8.4 at 4°C and 7.4 at 37°C. Tris has poor buffering capacity below pH 7.5.
4. *Zwitterionic* buffers contain both negative and positive groups so do not readily penetrate membranes. They are now widely used in biological experiments and HEPES (N-2-hydroxyethylpiperazine-N'-2-ethanesulphonic acid) is particularly useful. Its pK_a is 7.6.

NORMALITY–MOLARITY CONCEPT

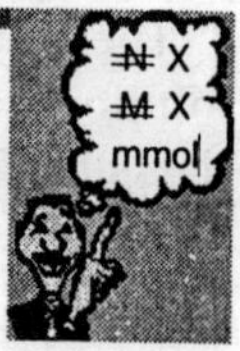

Molar Solutions

Molar solutions contain 1gm molecular weight of the solute/L of solution. 1 molar solution of H_2SO_4 contains 98.08 gm H_2SO_4/L (Mol W of H_2SO_4 = 98.08).

Normal Solutions

Normal solutions contain 1gm equivalent weight of the solute/L of solution. 1 mole HCl, 0.5 mole H_2SO_4, 0.333 mole H_3PO_4 in 1000 ml of solution in water are one normal solution. No. of moles × valency = No. of equivalents; molarity × valency = normality. The following equations define the expression of concentrations,

$$\text{Molarity of a solution} = \frac{\text{No. of moles of solute}}{\text{No. of liters of solution}}$$

$$\text{Normality of a solution} = \frac{\text{No. of gm equivalents of solute}}{\text{No. of litres of solution}}$$

The units of measure commonly used to express the concentrations of electrolytes in plasma is milliequivalents (mEq)/L or millimoles (mmol)/L.

$$\textbf{No. of mEq} = \frac{\text{Mass (g)} \times 1000}{\text{equivalent weight (g)}} = \frac{\text{Mass (g)} \times 1000 \times \text{valency}}{\text{MW}}$$

$$\textbf{No. of mmol} = \frac{\text{Mass (g)} \times 1000}{\text{MW}}$$

mg/100 ml can be converted to mEq/ L or mmol/ L as follows:

$$\text{mEq/ L} = \frac{\text{mg/100 ml} \times 10 \times \text{valency}}{\text{atomic or molecular mass}}$$

$$\text{mmol/ L} = \frac{\text{mg/ 100 ml} \times 10}{\text{atomic or molecular mass}}$$

Example: If serum sodium is 322 mg/ 100 ml [3220 mg/ L].
Atomic wt. of Na = 23, Valency = 1
mEq/ L = (322 × 10 × 1)/ 23 =140
Sodium concentration in plasma is also expressed as mmol/ L.

5

Centrifugation

Principle

Centrifugation is a technique used for the separation of particles using a centrifugal field. The particles suspended in liquid medium are placed in a centrifuge tube. The tube is then placed in a rotor and spun at a definitive speed. Rotation of the rotor about a central axis generates a specific centrifugal force upon the particles in the suspension.

Two forces counteract the centrifugal force acting on the suspended particles:

i. *Buoyant force*: This is the force with which the particles must displace the liquid media into which they sediment.

ii. *Frictional force*: This is the force generated by the particles as they migrate through the solution.

Particles move away from the axis of rotation in a centrifugal field only when the centrifugal force exceeds the counteracting buoyant and frictional forces resulting in sedimentation of the particles at a constant rate.

Centrifugal Field

Particles which differ in density, size or shape sediment at different rates. The rate of sedimentation depends upon:

1. The applied centrifugal field
2. Density and radius of the particle.
3. Density and viscosity of the suspending medium.

Angular velocity = ω radians/second; since one revolution = 360° = 2π radians

$$\text{One revolution/minute} = \text{rpm} = \frac{\omega \times 60}{2\pi}$$

$$\omega = \frac{2\pi \times (\text{rpm})}{60}$$

Therefore,

$$\text{Centrifugal field } (\mathbf{CF}) = \omega^2 \times r = \frac{[2\pi \times (\text{rpm})]^2}{[60]^2} \times r$$

$$= \frac{4\,\pi^2 \times (\text{rpm})^2 \times r}{3600}$$

(r = radial distance of the particle from the axis of rotation)

As the centrifugal field acting on the particle is much greater than the Earth's gravitational field, CF is generally expressed relative to the Earth's gravitational field as multiples of g, the acceleration due to gravity ($g = 980\ cm/s^2$)

$$\textit{Relative centrifugal field}\ (\text{RCF}) = \frac{\omega^2 \times r}{g}$$

$$\text{RCF} = \frac{4\,\pi^2 \times (\text{rpm})^2}{600 \times 980} \times r = 1.11 \times 10^{-5} \times (\text{rpm})^2 \times r$$

This expression relates relative centrifugal field (RCF) to the speed of the centrifuge (rpm) and the radius of the rotor (r). For example, if a rotor with an average radius of 7 cm revolves at a speed of 20,000 rpm, a centrifugal field of 31,300 g is created.

Sedimentation Coefficient

The sedimentation rate of velocity (v) of a particle can be expressed in terms of its sedimentation rate per unit centrifugal field. This is termed as sedimentation coefficient (s). The sedimentation rate is proportional to ω^2 r, the centrifugal field,

$v = s\,\omega^2\, r$

$$\text{Therefore, } s = \frac{v}{\omega^2 r}$$

Sedimentation velocity depends upon the mass of the particle, its density, shape and also on the density and viscosity of the medium in which the particle is suspended.

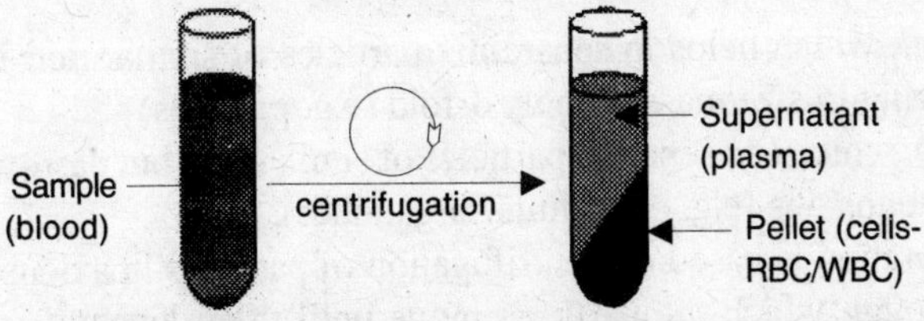

Fig.5.1: A simplified representation of a centrifugation cycle of a biological sample

Types of Centrifuges

	Low speed	*High speed*	*Ultracentrifuge*
1. Speed range (rpm)	2000-10000	18000-30000	40000-100000
2. Refrigeration	Some	Yes	Must
3. Vacuum system	None	Some	Must
4. Application for pelleting			
Cells	Yes	Yes	Yes
Nuclei	Yes	Yes	Yes
Membranous organelles	–	Yes	Yes
Membrane	–	Some	Yes
Ribosome or polysome	–	–	Yes
Macromolecules	–	–	Yes

The low speed centrifuge is commonly used in the clinical laboratory to separate serum or plasma from whole blood and also in deproteination of physiological fluids.

Types of Centrifugal Separation

Differential Centrifugation

This method is based on the differences in the sedimentation rate of particles of different size and density. The heaviest particles sediment first and by increasing the speed or time the lighter particles also pellet down. For particles with the same mass but different densities, the separation depends on density. Particles with higher density sediment first. For particles of similar densities, their separation can be achieved if their mass differs at least 10-fold from each other. This technique can help isolate the major cellular compartments.

Density Gradient Centrifugation

Centrifugation is carried out in a medium with a viscous gradient or density gradient. There are two techniques of density gradient centrifugation:

a. *rate zonal*, which helps in separating particles of similar density, but differing in size/mass by only 3-fold (e.g. proteins)
b. *isopycnic*, which can separate particles of similar size but narrowly different densities (e.g. subcellular organelles).

This separation is based on centrifugation of particles in a density gradient through which the particles move until their density is the same as that of the surrounding medium.

Types of Rotors

There are four main types of rotors for preparative centrifuges. They are swing bucket, fixed angle, vertical and zonal rotors.

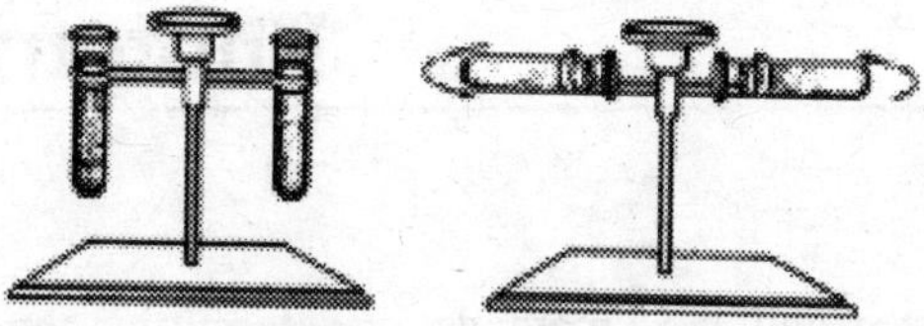

Fig. 5.2: A simple swing bucket rotor representation

Precautions

1. It is important that the tubes/centrifuge cups in the rotor head be balanced before centrifugation. This will permit maximum RCF and minimize breakage of tubes, wear on the motor and bearings and loss of sample.
2. Tubes should be properly capped and the lid of thc centrifuge should be closed during centrifugation. This will prevent the release of infectious material inside the centrifuge by aerosol formation. If breakage occurs resulting in the spillage of potentially infectious material the centrifuge bowl will be contaminated. Spillage of the sample can lead to corrosion of the centrifuge. Therefore in case of any spillage, the centrifuge should be properly decontaminated and cleaned.

6

Photometry

Probably the most widely used methods for determining the concentration of biochemical compounds are photometry and colorimetry, which make use of the property that when light passes through a colored solution, some wavelengths are absorbed more than others giving a plot of the absorption spectrum of the compound in solution. The light that is not absorbed is transmitted through the solution and gives the solution its color. Much of photometry is based on two laws:

When a parallel beam of monochromatic light passes through a solution in a transparent vessel, the absorbance (A) of the solution is directly proportional to concentration (c) of the compound in the solution. This is *Beer's law.*

When monochromatic light passes through an absorbing medium its intensity decreases exponentially as the length of the absorbing medium increases. Therefore, absorbance is directly proportional to the thickness or length of the light path (l) through the solution. This is *Lambert's law.*

$A \propto c$ (Beer's law) ———————— 1

$A \propto l$ (Lambert's law) ———————— 2

By combining (1) and (2), we get $A = \varepsilon_{\lambda}\, c\, l$

Where ε, the proportionality constant is termed the *molar absorption coefficient*. It is specific for a given substance at a given wavelength. It is the absorbance of a one molar solution of a substance with a light path of one centimeter (if c is expressed in mol/L). But Beer's law applies to only dilute solutions and in practice the concentrations of the solutions that are used in photometry are usually in the mmol/ L range. In colorimetry, the absorption coefficient is not usually used. Concentration of an unknown solution can be determined by using equation 1, which is derived as follows:

Absorbance of test sample (A_t) = ε × concentration of test (C_t) × l

Absorbance of standard sample (A_s) = $\varepsilon \times$ concentration of standard (C_s) $\times$ 1

Hence, Conc. of test (C_t)

$$C_t = \frac{\text{Absorbance of test sample } (A_t)}{\text{Absorbance of standard sample } (A_s)} \times \text{Conc. of standard } (C_s)$$

The light path, l, is usually kept constant in photometric measurements at 1 cm. This is the diameter of the vessel (called the cuvette) containing the solution.

Photometric instruments measure transmittance which is defined as follows:

$$\text{Transmittance, T} = \frac{\text{Intensity of the emergent (or transmitted) light}}{\text{Intensity of the incident light}} = \frac{I_e}{I_o}$$

Transmittance is usually expressed on a range of 0 to 100%.

This is not very convenient since a plot of percent transmittance against concentration gives a negative exponential curve. So a term absorbance is defined so that it is dirctly proportional to the concentration of the substance

$$\text{Absorbance, A} = \log \frac{1}{T} = \log \frac{I_o}{I_e}$$

Absorbance has no units. Photometric instruments electronically convert the measured transmittance to absorbance values.

Limitations of Beer-Lambert law To obtain linearity of absorption versus concentration plot the following conditions have to be fulfilled

1. Light must be of narrow wave length and preferably monochromatic.
2. The wavelength at which maximum absorption is called the absorption maximum (λ max) of that compound. Measurement should be made at this wavelength.
3. There must be no ionization, association, dissociation or salvation of the solute with concentration or time.
4. The law only holds good upto a threshold maximum concentration for a given substance. Hence, the solution should not be too concentrated.

A *standard* (or calibrator) is representative of the substance whose concentration is sought to be determined. The concentration of the compound in the test sample is obtained by comparing its absorbance with that of a known concentration of a standard solution. Ideally, a series of standards of known concentration are prepared to obtain a standard (calibration) curve. This helps to determine the range of concentrations over which Beer's law is obeyed.

Absorption spectra Many compounds have characteristic absorption spectra in the UV or visible regions so that their identification in a mixture is possible.

Proteins absorb strongly at 280 nm according to their content of the amino acids tyrosine, phenglalanine and tryptophan. Proteins absorb in the far UV due to the peptide bond.

Nucleic acids show maximum absorption around 260 nm. The extent of absorption is a measure of nucleic acid integrity since partially degraded acids absorb more strongly than the native material.

Hemoproteins absorb in visible as well as UV range due to the heme group. Characteristic shifts of the absorption maxima occurs when hemoglobin interacts with O_2, CO or drugs, so modified forms can be detected and measured.

Colorimetry

Colorimetry uses the basic principles of photometry but the solutions have to be colored, i.e. they must absorb light in the visible range. Colorless compounds are converted into colored compounds using chemical reactions. Under defined reaction conditions, the quantity of color formed is proportional to the quantity of the original colorless compound, hence using a simple colorimeter, estimation of amount of many compounds can be performed. This technique is unarguably the most widely used technique in medical biochemistry and almost every estimation protocol makes use of it.

Spectrofluorimetry

When a molecule after absorbing radiation, emits radiation of a longer wavelength, the phenomenon is called fluorescence. The increase, in wavelength is known as the Stoke's shift. Absorption of photons leads to excitation of electrons in less than 10^{-15} seconds. The energy emitted from these molecules in regaining the ground state within a period of less than 10^{-8} seconds gives rise to a fluorescent peak.

The requirements for fluorescence are an absorbing structure and high resonance energy. At low concentrations the intensity of fluorescence (I_f) is related to the incident radiation (I_o) as follows:

$$I_f = 2.3\, I_o\, \varepsilon_\lambda\, c\, d\, Q$$

Where,

ε = molar absorption coefficient for the absorbing material at wavelength λ,

c = concentration of the fluorescing solution

d = light path in the fluorescing solution

Q = quantum efficiency, the ratio of the quanta fluoresced to the quanta absorbed, which is independent of the exciting wavelength.

That is, $I_f \propto c$, fluorescence intensity is directly related to concentration. Spectrofluorimetry is most accurate at very low concentrations, in the picogram range, where spectrophotometry is least accurate. It enables the utilization of great spectral selectivity since due to Stoke's shift two monochromators are used, one selecting for the activating wavelength and the other the fluorescing wavelength.

The disadvantages of spectrofluorimetry include its susceptibility to pH, temperature and solvent polarity. Quenching is a major problem with fluorimetry where the energy absorbed is transferred to adjacent molecules. Though in some cases, the quenching reaction is specific enough for the identification of a fluorescent compound.

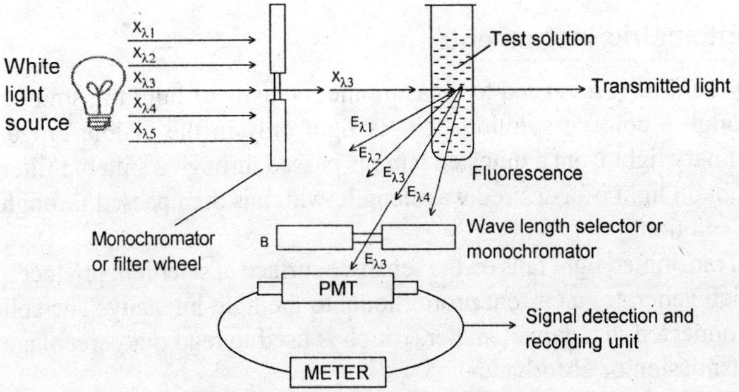

Where, $X_{\lambda3}$ is the excitation wavelength (Excitation maxima) $E_{\lambda3}$ is the emission wavelength (Emission maxima) for the test compound

Fig. 6.1: Working of a spectrofluorimeter

Applications

Identification of Compounds

a. Intrinsic fluorescence spectra of native compounds aid in their identification.
b. Non-fluorescent compounds can be detected by coupling to a fluorescent probe or fluor. For example, ethidium bromide or acridine orange can be linked to DNA, amino acids and peptides may be detected by coupling their primary amino groups to Dansyl chloride.

Quantitative Analysis

Assays of vitamins such as B_1, NADH, hormones like cortisol and estradiol, drugs such as barbiturates, pesticides, porphyrins and metal ions can be done accurately and with high sensitivity. Fluorescent dyes like Quin-2 and Fura-2 can be used for calcium studies.

Enzyme Assays

Conversion of NADH and NADPH to NAD^+ and $NADP^+$ can be monitored.

Fluorescence Bleaching Recovery

This is a technique for studying the motion of specific components in a complex mixture such as, fluorescently labeled phospholipids in biological membranes, e.g. diffusion of rhodopsin through photoreceptor membranes.

Photometric Instruments

Colorimeter. It is used to measure the intensity of light transmitted through a colored solution. It uses light only in the visible range. Ordinary light from a tungsten lamp is passed through a suitable filter to obtain light of a desired wavelength, which is then passed through the solution.

Transmitted light falls on the sensitive surface of selenium photocell which generates a current proportional to the light intensity. The cell is connected to a galvanometer, which is used to read out percentage transmission or absorbance.

Spectrophotometer. A spectrophotometer works on the same principle as a colorimeter but it is more sensitive and sophisticated.

There are light sources that emit light in the ultraviolet, visible and infrared regions of the spectrum. The wavelength is selected using a prism or diffraction grating and narrower bandwidths can be selected. Since light in the ultraviolet and infrared ranges is also emitted, the compound to be estimated does not necessarily have to be colored and can be measured directly if they significantly absorb even at these wavelengths. This offers a significant advantage over the colorimeter, which is restricted only in the visible range.

Types of Spectrophotometers

Grating spectrophotometers. In these spectrophotometers, the monochromator is a diffraction grating, which disperses the white light into a continuous spectrum. By turning the wavelength adjustment knob, the grating is rotated and different parts of the spectrum are allowed to fall on the photocell. In this manner, the desired wavelength can be selected.

Prism spectrophotometers. The prisms may be made of glass or quartz. Light from a tungsten filament is focused on the entrance slit and it passes through a glass prism that forms an extended spectrum. Only the light that falls on the exit slit can pass through the cuvette and illuminate the photocell. The monochromatic light obtained here is much more pure than that produced by light filters, i.e. a much narrower band of wavelength is present in the incident beam of light. Different photocells are used, one sensitive to the short wavelength range of the instrument (360-525 nm), while the other is used for the longer wavelengths (600 to 1000 nm). The total wavelength range at which measurements can be made includes the visible spectrum (400 to 700 nm) and extends on each side into the near ultraviolet (360 to 450 nm) and the near infrared (750 to 1000 nm). It is therefore possible to estimate substances that are more or less colorless in the visible region, but which absorb light in the ultraviolet or infrared regions. Quartz prisms help in extending the wavelength range below 350 nm down to about 190 nm. A deuterium lamp with a quartz envelope is provided as an additional light source. This is a rich source of UV radiation. Quartz cuvette will also be needed if one has to work in the UV range.

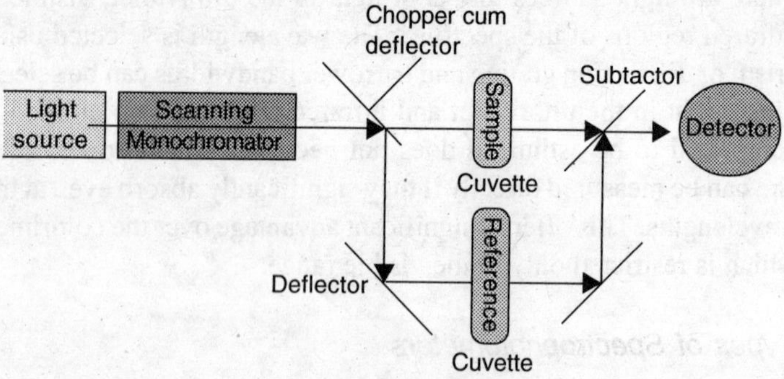

Fig. 6.2: Working of a double beam spectrophotometer

Uses. A spectrophotometer can be used for routine analysis in clinical chemistry. By using a narrower bandwidth than what is available with ordinary filters, the absorbance is often higher and the relation between absorbance and concentration remains linear over a wide range. If very dilute color is to be measured (e.g. in serum iron determinations), then a spectrophotometer is usually required. Analytical methods depending on ultraviolet absorption are commonly used in clinical chemistry and research. Examples include serum enzyme assays, assays of glucose, urea, uric acid, etc. which take advantage of the UV absorption of the coenzymes NADH and NADPH at 340 nm. For such methods a quartz spectrophotometer is essential.

ELISA reader. ELISA stands for "enzyme-linked immunosorbent assay." The ELISA reader or microplate reader is a modification of the colorimeter, which enables quantitation of upto 96 samples per microplate. Microplates have a 12 × 8 well format. A set of 8 lamps, 8 filters and 8 detectors enable the sequential determination of 96 samples.

Flowcytometer. Different populations of molecules, cells or particles can be differentiated by size and shape using forward and right angle light scatter. These cell particles or molecules can be labeled with different fluorescent labels or with dye labeled monoclonal antibodies. In this way, we can measure the amounts or isolate individual cells or populations of particular cells from a mixed population.

In flowcytometry, cells are made to flow in a single cell stream in a flow cell by hydrodynamic focussing. In hydrodynamic focussing, the sample stream containing the cells (of fixed wavelength, e.g.; argon laser gas wavelength of 488 nm) of sheath fluid. A laser is focussed on the cells. Various sensors pick up the laser light reflected by the cells.

The parameters measured by the flowcytometer are:

1. Forward scatter (FS)-FS is a measure of cellular size.
2. Side scatter (SS)-SS is measure of the granularity of the cell.
3. Fluorescence sensors (FL1-FL8).

The FL sensors measure light emitted by various dyes bound to the cells. The emitted light is directed into various sensors by a combination of filters. The commonly used dyes are fluorescein isothiocyanate (FITC), rhodamine (RD) and propidium iodide (PI). Fluorescence compensation is carried out to correct the overlaps in emission spectra of the fluorescent dyes. The measured data is displayed as one-parameter histograms, two parameter dot-plots or contour-plots. Regions defined in these plots are referred to as gates.

Fluorescence activated cell sorter (FACS) This is an advanced version of a flowcytometer, which uses an electrostatic field to separate cells with preselected fluorescence characteristics into two reservoirs on the basis of polarity and quantity of charge. Unselected cells in uncharged droplets fall into another tube.

A simplified line diagram illustrating FACS and cell sortor operation (Fig. 6.3).

Applications. As multiple parameters-size, granularity, DNA or RNA content, DNA nucleotide ratios, cellular antigens and receptors, etc. can be measured using these instruments, they have come to be used widely in research and applied medicine.

For example counting of blood cells including differential counting of leukocytes, isolating T cell subsets, tissue typing, in diagnosis, treatment and prognosis in cancer, in study of the cell cycle and apoptosis, karyotyping, diagnosis of bacterial infections, etc.

Automated clinical chemistry analyzers. These usually incorporate mechanized versions of basic manual laboratory techniques and procedures. They help in the processing, transport and testing of a large number of clinical specimens in an efficient manner. Work is simplified by using robotic and computer technology to undertake repetitive tasks like pipetting, dispensing and mixing. Advanced

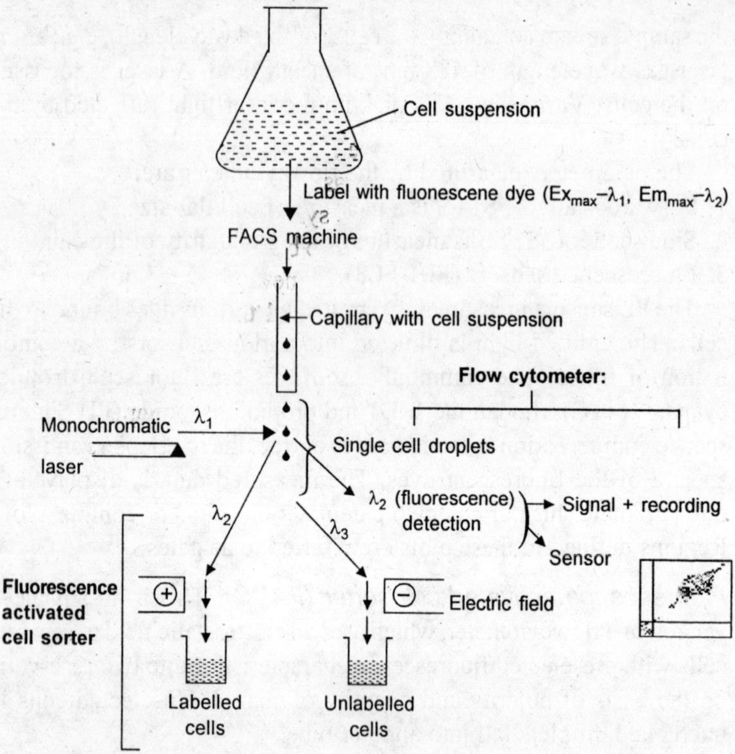

Fig. 6.3: A simplified line diagram illustrating FACS and cell sorter operation

versions of the spectrophotometer help in increasing specimen throughout.

Precautions

1. *Care of cuvettes* Soak in 50% v/v nitric acid and then rinse with distilled water. Check cuvettes against each other for small differences in optical properties. Always wipe the outside of the cuvettes with soft tissue paper before placing in the cell holder. Do not handle them by the optical faces. After use, rinse with distilled water.

2. *Absorption of radiation by cuvettes* Absorption of radiation by cuvettes occurs at different wavelengths depending upon the

material from which it is made. Expensive silica cuvettes, which are most transparent to UV, are used in the far UV. Glass cuvettes, which absorb in UV range and cannot be used below 360 nm, are used in the visible region. Plastic cuvettes, which absorb UV less than glass, can be used conveniently at 340 nm.

3. *Light source* For a broad range of radiations tungsten lamp is used, whereas for UV deuterium lamp is used. To use tungsten lamp at 360-400 nm, a blue filter is placed in the light beam.

4. *Blanks* Appropriate blanks are used to exclude the absorbance contributed by the solvents and reagents, i.e. by everything other than the compound of interest.

7

Radioactivity

Radioactive isotopes are unstable atomic species, which disintegrate to form stable isotopes. During disintegration, they emit particles and/or electromagnetic radiation due to changes in the composition of the atomic nucleus. These processes are known as radioactive decay and could involve emission of alpha particles or negatrons or gamma rays. Some of the commonly used radioactive isotopes include ^{3}H, ^{32}P, ^{35}S and ^{131}I. The advantage of using isotopes in biochemistry is that they specifically label molecules without altering their chemical properties. Isotope effects, which are changes in reaction rates arising from mass differences between isotopes, are generally negligible. They have consequently become labels of choice over chemical labeling techniques and process. The process of radioactive decay leads to emission of particles with the following characteristic energies.

Alpha Particles (α)

They are double charged helium nuclei and are emitted by high atomic number radioactive elements. These radiations do not penetrate skin and hence are not severely toxic. But repeated exposure of same area to body to α-emitters can lead to tissue injury which might develop into cancer. The α-emitters are not so commonly used in research.

Beta Radiation (β)

Emitted by most commonly used radioactive isotopes in research like ^{32}P, ^{3}H, ^{14}C. It essentially comprises high speed electrons (β^{-}) with a range of energies. Whereas low energy radiations are absorbed by skin, the high energy radiations can penetrate skin and may lead to development of skin burns.

Gamma Radiation (γ)

Electromagnetic radiation of short wavelength without any mass or charge and hence extremely penetrating, forms areas of ionization after collisions with various atoms. Some isotopes which emit gamma–radiations include ^{131}I and ^{54}Fe.

Radioactive Half Lives

Radioactive decay is a spontaneous and random process, the rate of which depends only on the number of radioactive atoms present. It is therefore a first order reaction whose half life, $t_{½}$, is a function only of the rate constant k, for the decay process:

$$t_{½} = \frac{Ln\ 2}{k} = \frac{0.693}{k}$$

Since k, the rate constant is different for each isotope; each has a characteristically different half life. The characteristics of some commonly used isotopes are listed in Table 7.1.

Table 7.1: Properties of some commonly used radioisotopes

Isotope nucleus	*Radiation nature*	*Half life*
^{3}H	β	12.32 years
^{14}C	β	5715 years
^{32}P	β	14.28 days
^{35}S	β	87.2 days
^{60}Co	β, γ	5.217 years
^{125}I	γ	59.4 days
^{131}I	β, γ	8.04 days

Units in Radioactivity Measurement

The SI unit of radioactivity is the Becquerel (Bq) and it corresponds to one disintegration per second from a radioactive sample. Traditionally, radioactivity was measured in terms of Curie named after the Nobel laureate Madam Curie who discovered radium, hence Ci, which was originally defined as the activity of 1 gram of radium, later designated more precisely as 3.7×10^{10} disintegrations per second.

1 mCi = 37 MBq

1 MBq = 27 pCi

Technically it is not possible to detect disintegrations from the samples hence the terminology of 'counts per minute' is used to designate the strength of radioactivity.

Detection and Measurement of Radioactivity

Radioactive isotopes interact with matter in two ways, causing ionization and excitation. There are three commonly used methods of detecting and quantifying radioactivity. These are based on the ionization of gases, the ability of ionizing radioactivity to expose photographic emulsions, i.e. autoradiography, and excitation of solids or solutions.

Methods Based Upon Ionization (Proportional Counting)

As a charged particle passes through a gas, its electrostatic field dislodges orbital electrons from atoms sufficiently close to its path and causes ionization. α and β particles may be detected by gas ionization methods, but these methods are poor for detecting γ-radiation. Geiger-Muller counters are based on the ionization of gases. Though these counters are easy to use, two of the most commonly used radioisotopes ^{3}H and ^{14}C have insufficient penetration power to enter a proportional counter's detection chamber with reasonable efficiency.

Ionizing radiation acts upon a silver based photographic emulsion to produce a latent image as produced by visible light due to reduction of silver halide to metallic silver. For a photograph, a radiation source, an object to be imaged and photographic emulsion are required. For an autoradiograph, a radiation source (i.e. radioactivity) emanating from within the material of study (e.g. labeled proteins, metabolites, etc.) exposes the photographic film and leads to its blackening analogous to blackening by X-rays by deposition of metallic silver.

Methods Based Upon Excitation

Excitation leads the excitable compound (known as the fluorophore) to emit photons of light. This fluorescence can be detected and quantified. The process is known as scintillation and this light when detected by a photomultiplier tube, forms the basis of scintillation counting. The electric pulse that results from the conversion of light energy to electrical energy in the photomultiplier is directly proportional to the energy of the original radioactive event.

There are two types of scintillation counting.

i. *Solid counting.* In solid scintillation counting, the sample is placed adjacent to a crystal of fluorescent material. The crystal that is normally used for γ-isotopes is sodium iodide, whereas for α-emitters zinc sulphide crystals are preferred and for β-emitters organic scintillators such as anthracene are used. The crystals themselves are placed near to a photomultiplier tube, which in turn is connected to a high voltage supply and a scaler. Solid scintillation counting is particularly useful for γ-emitting isotopes (e.g. ^{131}I). This is because γ-rays are electromagnetic radiations and causes ionization or excitation of neighboring atoms. Conversely, solid scintillation counting is generally unsuitable for weak β-emitting isotopes.

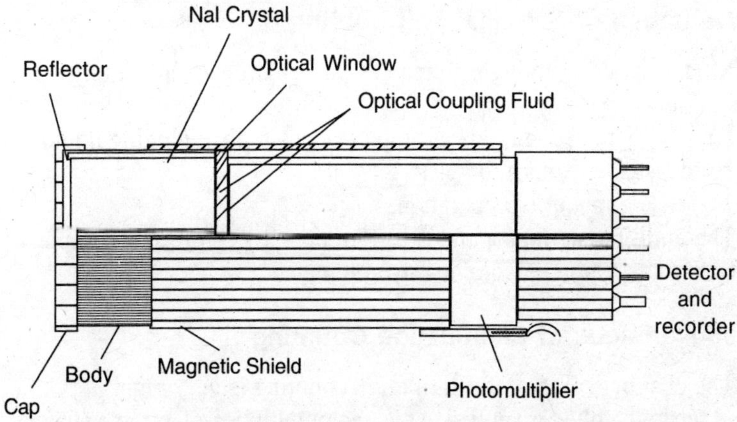

Fig. 7.1: Schematic representation of a solid scintillation counter

ii. *Liquid scintillation counting:* In liquid counting, the radioactive sample is mixed with scintillation cocktail containing one or more fluorophores (a chemical compound which emits a pulse of light when struck with a radiation). This method is useful in quantifying weak β-emitters such as ^{32}P, ^{3}H and ^{35}S. Since they are β-emitters, the energy is transferred to the organic solution, which is insufficient to be detected by photomultiplier tubes; hence a primary fluor is used to trap that energy. To increase the efficiency and detection sensitivity of the PMT a secondary fluor is used in the sample which shifts the wavelength of the emission close the detection range of photomultiplier tube. For example, toluene is used as the organic solvent to which energy from an emission is transferred, which transfers this energy to primary fluorophore PPO (2, 5–diphenyloxazole) which then transfers to the secondary fluorophore POPOP [1, 4-bis-(5–phenyloxazol-2-yl) benzene] which emits the radiation as a light emission of the visible range which can be effectively detected by PMT.

Besides these counting sometimes the radioactive samples are directly counted without the scintillation fluid. Such a process is called as Cerenkov counting and occurs because of ionization of air. This is possible only for strong β-emitting isotopes like ^{32}P, ^{42}K, etc. Though such a counting gives a fairly good estimation of radioactivity in the samples, it is not the accurate estimation of disintegrations per minute (dpm) from the samples.

Advantages of Scintillation Counting

1. Much higher counting efficiencies particularly for low energy β-emitters.
2. The ability to accommodate samples of any type, including liquids, solids, suspensions and gels.
3. The ease of sample preparation.
4. The ability to count separately different isotopes in same sample.
5. Scintillation counters are highly automated.

Disadvantages of Scintillation Counting

1. The cost per sample of scintillation counting is very high.
2. At the high voltages applied to the photomultiplier, electronic events occur in the system independent of radioactivity but contribute to a high background count.
3. Quenching
4. Chemiluminescence can also cause problems during liquid scintillation counting.
5. Phospholuminescence results from components of the sample, including the vial itself, absorbing light and re-emitting it.

Safety Aspects

The greatest disadvantage of using radioisotopes is their toxicity. They produce ionizing radiations which can cause severe sickness like dizziness, nauseous feeling and headache if exposed for high-dose for short duration, but leads to mutagenesis associated complications of various cells over long period of time. When handling radioisotopes the following preconditions should be met and the following precautions should be taken:

- Make a separate radioactivity handling and processing room, with clearly marked radiation hazard mark on the door and working space (Black symbol in yellow background on doors and working space and in orange background on the bottles carrying such reagents).

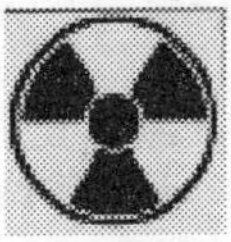

Fig. 7.2: On working space

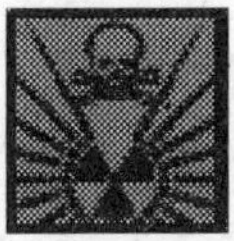

Fig. 7.3: On bottles/carriers, etc.

- Get proper authorization from the Board of Radiation and Isotope Technology (BRIT). They are authorized suppliers of radioactivity material for use in research in India.
- Procure the 'Exposure Dose estimation' film-badge from BRIT to monitor the exposure. The badge should be worn on the trunk or the wrist of the user at all times. A pocket dosimeter is helpful if strong α or β–emitters are used.
- Procure proper shields and maintain them at all times. The recommended prespex or lead shields should be used.
- Maximize the distance between yourself and the source as much as possible.
- Minimize the time of exposure of samples. Keep them behind shield or inside designated carriers at all times.
- Dispose the material properly and do not flush the material through the sink.

Use of Radioisotopes in Molecular Biology

The use of radioisotopes has revolutionized many aspects and areas of research. A few common applications are listed under:

1. Metabolic studies–Tracing a metabolic pathway have become a much simpler task after utilization of radiolabeled precursors in the pathway. Similarly, the drug catabolism pathway can be analysed using labeled progenitors.
2. In enzyme kinetics analysis.
3. Radioimmunoassays.

4. Radiodating.
5. Diagnostic applications–Kidney function test using ^{131}I, etc.
6. Molecular biology applications–For tagging DNA, RNA, proteins, etc.

Table 7.2: Radiation derived units

Quantity	*Old Unit*	*SI Unit*	*New Unit*	*Conversion*
Activity	curie (Ci)	disintegration per second	Becquerel	1 μCi = 37 GBq
Absorbed dose	rad	Joule per kilogram (J/kg)	gray (Gy)	1 Gy = 100 rad
Exposure	roentgen	Coulomb per kilogram (C/kg)	—	1 C/kg = 3798 R
Dose equivalent	rem	Joule per kilogram (J/kg)	sievert	1 Sv = 100 rem

8

Electrophoresis

Electrophoresis is the movement of charged particles through an electrolyte in an electric field. The positively charged particles move towards the cathode and the negative ions to the anode. The rate of migration of particles of like charge will depend among other things on the number of charges it carries. Different rates of migration separate a complex mixture such as plasma proteins into a number of fractions according to mobility. Electrophoresis has been used since long in research and clinical laboratories for fractionation of protein molecules.

Molecular biology techniques like Southern and Northern blotting, Polymerase Chain Reaction, restriction enzyme digestion and the cloning of DNA are becoming important diagnostic tools in the hands of physicians. In most of these techniques, fractionation of nucleic acids is an intigrat part and hence electrophoresis becomes a crucial component for everybody.

Types of Electrophoresis

The earliest form of electrophoresis (moving boundary) was carried out in free solution but mixing of components by convection currents proved a problem. Nowadays, electrophoresis is carried out on a supporting matrix and complete separation of a mixture can be effected into distinct zones. Some commonly used support media are:

Paper. Filter paper is cheap and easy to use. The main disadvantage is that some mixing occurs between the zones due to adsorption on the cellulose.

Cellulose acetate. Shows minimal adsorption and clear separation of a mixture into separate zones. Compounds are easily eluted with a good recovery. Very small sample is required and it takes only hours as compared to overnight for paper electrophoresis. However, cellulose acetate is more expensive than paper.

Agar-gel. Agar is transparent, making it suitable for photometric scanning. It is the material of choice for immunoelectrophoresis. Agar is cheap and readily available. Purified agar called as agarose is used specifically for separation of nucleic acids, as it forms the pores of very uniform size, hence giving highly reproducible and accurate resolution.

Starch. This medium is prepared by compressing whole starch grains in a buffer into a block. Large molecules are separated and it is ideal for separation and isolation of isozymes.

Polyacrylamide The major advantage is its transparency so that it can be scanned in visible and the UV. Fine resolution of complex mixtures is possible and the pore size can be controlled, so that separation can be on the basis of size and shape of the molecules as well as the charge.

Buffers in Electrophoresis

The suspension buffer has to be carefully selected since some buffer ions react with the compounds under investigation; borate, for example forms complexes with sugars while citrate and EDTA will chelate metal ions such as calcium.

The pH chosen depends on the particular mixture under investigation. Generally, the maximum separation is obtained at the isoelectric point of one of the compounds. The pH selected should not cause chemical changes or denaturation of the molecules under investigation.

The ionic strength of the buffer usually lies in the range 0.05-0.15. At low ionic strength, there is rapid migration and low heat production but marked diffusion. On the other hand, at high ionic strength sharp bands are obtained, but there is a higher heat production and migration is over a shorter distance.

Electrical Field

A stable d.c. source is required which gives a constant current or voltage. Field strength from 5 to 8 V/cm is suitable for most separations at room temperature. If the field strength is greater than 10 V/cm then the heating effect is such that an excessive amount of water is lost by evaporation. The buffer then flows from the buffer tanks to replace the water lost by evaporation which causes displacement of the zones.

If the heating is excessive, compounds may be denatured. Methods of cooling are available so that higher field strength can be used but special equipment with efficient cooling and a number of foolproof devices is needed for working with higher voltages. Such specialized high voltage equipment can be used successfully to resolve mixtures of low molecular weight compounds which suffer from excess diffusion thus the method needs to be very rapid. However, most common electrophoretic separations involve charged macromolecules where diffusion is minimal.

Polyacrylamide Gel Electrophoresis (PAGE)

The gel is prepared immediately before use from acrylamide ($CH_2 = CHCONH_2$) and a small quantity of cross-linking reagent, methylene bisacrylamide ($CH_2 = CHCONH)_2$ CH_2), in the presence of a catalyst accelerator-chain initiator mixture. This mixture consists of freshly prepared ammonium persulphate as catalyst (0.1 to 0.3% w/v) together with about the same concentration of a suitable base, e.g. dimethyl aminopropionitrile (DMAP) or tetramethylethylene-diamine (TEMED) as initiator.

The porosity of the gel is determined by relative proportion of acrylamide monomer with cross-linking agent. The gels may be defined in terms of total percentage of acrylamide present, 30% of gel is suitable for the separation of compounds having molecular weight around 10^4Da. and 3% for molecular weight around 10^6Da.

Features of polyacrylamide gel that makes it unique for gel electrophoresis:

a. Polyacrylamide gels have minimal adsorption capacity.
b. They lack electro-osmosis and their general stability for *in situ* quantitative analysis and various types of histochemical analysis.
c. The matrix is very flexible yet strong, thus permitting efficient handling.

Staining of Gels

A variety of stains are used:

a. *Coomassie Brilliant Blue (CBB)* It binds non-specifically to any protein; even at a low concentration of 1 μg. CBB is available in two forms: CBB-R_{250} and CBB-G_{250}. CBB-R_{250} is fast binding dye; it binds to proteins through SO^{3-} moieties present on it. In this type of staining, the extent of staining also determines the amount of protein in the gel.

b. *$CuCl_2$* This is used for negative staining. The gel takes up blue color and the protein remains colorless.

c. *KCl* Incubation of gel with 0.25 M KCl solution stains the gel off-white leaving resolved protein colorless. It is particularly useful when protein needs isolation from a mixture for immunization or activity studies.

d. *Silver staining* Highly sensitive staining; stains proteins even in the low concentration of 0.1 ng. Electrophoretically resolved proteins are fixed on gel with methanol and acetic acid and further enhancement of fixing is done by glutaraldehyde. The proteins are then reduced with DTT (dithiothreitol). To this reduced protein silver (Ag) binds and is developed as silvercarbonate protein complex by adding developer. Stained proteins show on gel as brown bands.

e. *Specific stains:*
   i. Glycoproteins: Using PAS (Per Iodic Schiff's) reagent.
   ii. Lipoproteins: Using Sudan black or NBT (nitro blue tetrazolium oxide) stain.

SDS-PAGE

SDS–PAGE is a modified PAGE where the proteins are denatured in the presence of SDS and a thiol reagent (2-mercaptoethanol) which breaks the complex protein into its constituent polypeptides; SDS binds in a constant weight ratio (1.4 g per 1g of protein) which completely masks the natural charge of the protein giving it a constant charge to mass ratio and thus all proteins migrate in polyacrylamide gel according to polypeptide size (molecular weight). Under these conditions, a graph of $\log_{10}$ polypeptide molecular mass and relative mobility (Rf) shows a straight line relationship.

A set of marker peptides whose molecular masses are known are electrophoresed and the distance migrated by each of them is used to construct a standard curve using which molecular weight of the polypeptides can be determined, based on their mobility in the same gel. For a given gel concentration the relationship between $\log_{10}$ molecular weight and relative mobility is linear over a limited range of molecular weights.

Maleated polypeptides, collagenous polypeptides and polypeptides with high proline content give abnormally high molecular weight by SDS-PAGE, since they are very basic or very acidic proteins.

Requirements

a. 30% Acrylamide-bisacrylamide solution (29.2 g acylamide and 0.8 g bis-acylamide in 100 ml solution)
b. Tris-HCl buffer (1.5 M Tris-HCl, pH 8.8; 0.5 M Tris-HCl, pH 6.8)
c. SDS (10% w/ v)
d. Tris-Glycine buffer (25 mM Tris, 250 mM glycine [pH 8.3] 0.1% [w/v] SDS)
e. APS (ammonium per sulphate 10% w/v)
f. TEMED
g. 3x Sample buffer/loading dye (150 mM Tris-HCl, pH 6.8, 2.5% β-mercaptoethanol, 3% SDS, 30% Glycerol; 0.3% bromo phenol blue).
h. 1% Coomassie Brilliant Blue R_{250} (in H_2O; CH_3OH; CH_3COOH; in a ratio of 5 : 4 : 1 respectively).
i. Electrophoresis equipment.
j. Vacuum drier.

Methodology (For mini-gel of 7.5 ml only)

Pouring the 15% resolving gel. To 2.5 ml of 30% acrylamide: bisacrylamide solution, 1.1 ml of H_2O, 1.5 M Tris (pH ~ 8.8), 0.05 ml of 10% SDS, 0.05 ml of 10% APS and 3 μl of TEMED are added and poured to 3/4th the length of the plate. The gel is over-layered with water to prevent oxidation.

Pouring the 5% stacking gel. Once the resolving gel is polymerized, the stacking gel is prepared as follows: To 0.498 ml of 30% acrylamide–bisacrylamide solution, 2.04 ml of H_2O, 0.378 ml of 0.5 M Tris (pH ~ 6.8), 0.03 ml of 10% SDS, 0.03 ml of APS and 3 μl of TEMED are added and the gel poured over the separating/ resolving gel. The comb is adjusted immediately and the gel allowed to polymerize.

Running a 15% SDS PAGE gel. 20 μl of the sample is mixed with 10 μl of 3x SDS–PAGE loading dye/buffer and the mixture is incubated at 94°C for 5 minutes. The samples are then centrifuged and loaded in the wells/slots of the stacking gel and resolved at 25 mA till the BPB dye reaches the end of the separating gel.

Coomassie staining of gel. The resolved gel is carefully removed and transferred to Coomassie brilliant blue stain and kept shaking at room temperature for 15 to 20 minutes after a brief heating on microwave for 1 minute. Then the gel is transferred to destaining solution (Distilled water, acetic acid and methanol mixed in the ratio 60:10:30), which is kept shaking until the bands came up sharply against an almost clear background.

Gels can be dried later using vacuum drier.

Precautions. Acrylamide is toxic and should be handled with care; avoid skin contact.

Agarose Gel Electrophoresis of DNA

If a DNA molecule in solution is subjected to electrophoresis, it will migrate towards the anode due to the presence of the negatively charged phosphate groups. However, as there is one phosphate for every base, the charge per unit length of DNA is the same and so separation does not take place based on charge. Both sizes as well as the shape of the molecules influence resolution of DNA fragments. Larger molecules will experience more friction and be more retarded by the gel pores than the smaller molecules. Similarly, circular DNA (e.g. plasmids) will move faster than the linear DNA fragments.

The following factors influence the migration of DNA through agarose gel:

1. The molecular size of the DNA
2. The conformation of the DNA
3. The concentration of agarose
4. The applied voltage
5. Ionic composition of the electrophoresis buffer

Agarose gels, which have relatively larger pore size, are most suitable for the separation of DNA because routinely analyzed DNA molecules are considerably large. Agarose, a polygalactan, is purified from agar, which is a long-chain polysaccharide extracted from seaweed. Size of DNA is expressed in terms of the number of base pairs. Even a small fragment of DNA of the size of 1 kb (1000 base pairs) has a molecular weight of 620 kDa. The gel matrix can vary from 0.3-3% agarose (0.8 or 1% gels are used routinely) which can resolve DNA fragments from 60 kb to 0.2 kb. Polyacrylamide gels are used to separate DNA fragments less than 1kb. For instance, in sequencing DNA, fragments that differ in size by one nucleotide are resolved.

DNA that has separated in the gel according to size can be visualized by ethidium bromide staining. The dye intercalates between the bases and emits orange-red fluorescence under UV light. Silver staining yields red/ brown to brown/ black DNA bands in polyacrylamide gels.

Since agarose gel electrophoresis separates DNA according to size, the length of a DNA molecule can be determined by running a standard DNA marker of known molecular weight and length on the same gel. This is most conveniently achieved by running a sample of bacteriophage lambda DNA that has been cleaved with a restriction enzyme such as *Hind* III or *Eco*R I.

Methodology

1. To 400 mg of agarose taken in a glass conical flask 50 ml of TBE (Tris-borate-EDTA) buffer, pH 7.4, is added (final conc. of agarose is 0.8%) [TAE (Tris-acetate-EDTA) buffer can also be used]. Volume of the gel required depends on the size of the gel casting tray. The gel casting tray is sealed with adhesive tape on two sides and the comb is fitted to it.
2. The agarose solution is heated to boiling until all the particles have gone into solution and then poured in the casting tray and allowed to set (approx. 30 mins. at room temp).
3. After the gel is set, the tape is removed and the gel is wrapped in cling film along with a little amount of TBE buffer and stored refrigerated till further use.
4. 4 μl of 6 × loading dye (20% glycerol, 0.25% bromophenol blue and 0.25% xylene cyanol) is added to the previously digested 20 μl standard and test DNA samples (approx. 1 μg DNA).
5. 24 μl of this sample is loaded. The gel is run at 60-80 V until the bromophenol blue has moved sufficiently into the gel (half the gel length).
6. The gel is stained in 250 ml of ethidium bromide (10 μg/ml) in TBE buffer for 15 mins. and destained in double distilled water for 5 minutes. after which it is visualized on the UV transilluminator.

7. Migration of each band is measured and log size versus distance migrated in standard lane is plotted. The size of the test band can be read from the graph, using the distance migrated.
8. The presence or absence of normal expected band(s) or altered size of the band(s) is then used to interpret different diagnostic tests.

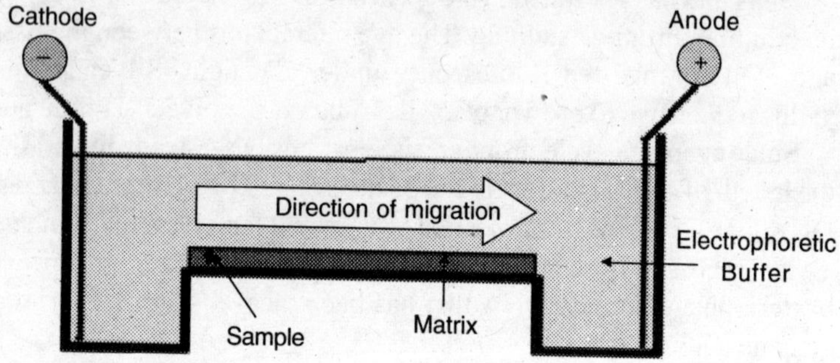

Fig. 8.1: Overview of a electrophoretic cell

Precautions

Ethidium bromide is a strong mutagen and therefore should be handled with utmost care, using gloves. Gels are quite fragile and liable to breakage. Handle them gently. While visualizing gels stained with EtBr do not expose eyes to UV light. Visualige gels with proper equipment and shields only.

9

Chromatography

The term 'Chromatography' means separation of colored compounds. This technique was originally used to separate chlorophyll from plant extracts on silica. Now, it is the name given to any technique in which the members of a group of similar substances are separated by a continuous redistribution between two phases based on differences in size, shape, mass, charge, solubility and adsorption properties. The stationary phase may be solid, liquid, gel or solid/liquid mixture which is immobilized. The second mobile phase may be liquid or gaseous and flows over or through the stationary phase. The choice of stationary or mobile phases is made so that the compounds to be separated have different distribution coefficients.

The movement of any substance being chromatographed is the outcome of:

a. Forces resulting from its interaction with the mobile phase which tend to pull it along with the mobile phase.
b. Forces resulting from its attraction to the stationary phase, which tend to retard its movement.

Since the forces are different for different substances chromatography will be able to separate out the components of a mixture of substances. Based on the properties of the stationary phase and the acting forces, several different types of chromatographic procedures have been described.

1. *Adsorption chromatography*: Adsorption equilibrium between a stationary solid and a mobile liquid phase, e.g. steroid separation.
2. *Partition chromatography*: Partition equilibrium between a stationary liquid and a mobile liquid phase.
3. *Gas-liquid chromatography*: Partition equilibrium between a stationary liquid and a mobile gaseous phase, e.g. steroid separation.
4. *Ion-exchange chromatography*: on exchange equilibrium between an ion-exchange stationary resin phase and a mobile electrolyte phase, e.g. protein separation.

5. *Gel permeation chromatography*: Equilibrium between a liquid phase inside and outside a porous molecular sieve depending on molecular size. It is essentially a preparative procedure.
6. *Affinity chromatography*: Equilibrium between a macromolecule and a small molecule (Ligand) for which it has high affinity, e.g. monoclonal antibody purification, affinity purification of proteins.

Paper Chromatography

Experiment

Amino acid separation by paper chromatography.

Principle. The amino acids partition themselves on the Whatman paper (1 or 3 MM) between an organic solvent of choice and water adsorbed between the cellulose fibers (stationary hydrophilic phase). For the separation of lipids and other hydrophobic molecules, silica impregnated papers are commercially available.

Methodology

There are two techniques, which may be employed for the development of paper chromatograms: ascending or descending methods.

In ascending technique, the paper is kept in a glass jar containing the solvent such that the lower edge of the paper is in contact with the solvent.

1. The sample is applied to the position just above the surface of the solvent.
2. As the solvent moves vertically up the paper by capillary action, separation of the amino acids is achieved. In the descending techniques, the solvent moves downwards under gravity.
3. Component detection: Spraying of the paper with ninhydrin will stain amino acids.
4. The identification of a given amino acid may be on the basis of its relative fraction. (R_f) value which is defined as:

$$R_f = \frac{\text{The distance moved by solute front}}{\text{The distance moved by solvent front}}$$

This value is constant for a particular compound under standard conditions.

7. Quantification of the amino acid may be carried out after eluting it with a suitable solvent.

Clinical Applications

1. Screening and diagnosis of inherited disorders of amino acid metabolism, e.g. phenylketonuria and tyrosinemia.
2. Peptide fingerprinting for the diagnosis of diseases like sickle cell anemia.
3. One-dimensional thin layer chromatography (TLC) can detect aminoacidopathies and is the most adequate for screening.

Specimens reference solution (mixture of known amino acids at known concentration) and controls are applied to thin layer plates, run in an appropriate solvent-vapor system and then dried and stained with ninhydrin.

Some solid matrices used in chromatoghraphic techniques. Dextran (Sephadex), agarose (Sepharose), silica gel and cellulose (Sephacel) are some of the solid support media for chromatography.

Gel Filtration

Principle. In the column, proteins of different molecular size penetrate into the internal pores of the beads to different degrees and thus travel down the column at different rates. In other words, very large protein molecules cannot enter the pores of the beads and they are excluded, while small proteins can enter the pores of the beads freely and are retarded. This is called molecular sieving or gel permeation. The different peaks of separation can be monitored by UV detectors and recorded. The peak containing required material can be identified depending upon the properties of the substance, e.g. measurement of enzyme activity, Ag-Ab binding, etc.

- *Exclusion limit:* Exclusion limit of a gel is the molecular weight of the smallest molecule incapable of penetrating the gel pores.
- *Bed volume(Vt)*: Volume of the gel which is available to those molecules which are smaller than the fractionation range for the gel.
- *Void volume (Vo):* Volume of the liquid in the interstitial spaces between beads of the gel. It is available to those molecules whose size is bigger than the fractionation range of the gel.
- *Stationery volume (Vx):* Volume of the solid matrix in the column.

$$Vt = Vo + Vx$$

- *Elution volume (Ve):* Amount of solution exiting from the column between the time the solute first penetrates the surface of column and it appears in the effluent. It is measured from the half maximum peak height of the leading edge.
- *Partition distribution coefficient (k_d)* = $\frac{Ve - Vo}{Vx}$

Experiment

Separation using G-50 Sephadex column of Hemoglobin- $K_2Cr_2O_7$ mixture.

Requirements.

1. Sephadex G-50 beads (Dextran is a polysaccharide) built from glucose residues. When the dextran is cross-linked by epichlorhydrin to form a gel, the polysaccharide chains of the gel from a three-dimensional network. The product is insoluble unless it is broken down chemically. Dextran gels are commercially known by the name of Sephadex. The different types of Sephadex beads differ in their degree of cross-linking. The various types are characterized by the letter G, followed by a number. Based on their extent of cross- linkage, proteins of different MW are separated from each other).
2. Phosphate buffered saline (PBS) 0.1 M pH 7.2.
3. Hemoglobin.
4. Potassium dichromate.

Methodology

1. In the provided columns of 0.8 cm × 24 cm pack, Sephadex G-50 used for fractionation of peptides and globular proteins in the range of 1000-5000 MW.
2. The gel was previously swollen in 1% ammonium hydroxide for 48 hours. To support the gel glass wool is used at the bottom. No air bubble should be there in the column and gel should never get dry.
3. Equilibrate column with PBS and adjust flow rate to 1 ml/2 mins.
4. Load 1 ml of the mixture of Hemoglobin (5 mg/ml) and $K_2Cr_2O_7$ (1 mg/ml) carefully on top of the column.
5. 1 ml fractions are collected; total fractions exceeding the bed volume of the column.
6. Absorbance 420 nm and 370 nm (λ max for hemoglobin and dichromate respectively) taken for each fraction.

7. A combined graph having peaks of both the wavelengths plotted.
8. Using the graph elution volume for both the compounds is calculated.

Since Sephadex G-50 has a fractionation range of 1000-5000 Da, Hemoglobin which has a molecular weight of 64,000 Da comes in the void volume and is eluted initially, whereas $K_2Cr_2O_7$ which has a molecular weight of 200 Da enters the beads of Sephadex, thus is eluted later beyond void volume but within bed volume.

Thin Layer Chromatography (TLC)

Thin layer chromatography employs application of matrix meant for separation, as a thin layer, on which chromatography is performed. Any substance that can be finely divided and can be formed into thin slurry can be used as matrix. TLC is meant exclusively for the separation of small molecules.

Sample applied on the thin layer are separated with a developing solvent, where the components are separated on the basis of following factors

A. *Partition:* partition equilibrium between the stationary phase and mobile liquid phase separates the components of a mixture based on their partition coefficients

$$Kd = \frac{\text{Concentration in phase A}}{\text{Concentration in phase B}}$$

B. *Adsorption:* Depending upon the extent of specific interaction between the sample components and the stationary phase (matrix), components get adsorbed or fail to do so. Depending upon the solubility in the mobile phase solvent, components are retarded in their movement.

Experiment

The separation of lipids using TLC.

Principle Lipids in biological material are present as a complex mixture and are first fractionated into a number of groups by solvent extraction. Resolution of the compounds within each group can then be carried out by TLC. The solvent is selected according to the lipids under investigation. Generally, neutral lipids are separated with a non-polar solvent and charged lipids with polar solvents. Silica gel has been widely used for separation of lipids based on adsorption as well as partition, even though there are also a number of other supporting media that can be used.

In this experiment, lipids are separated into groups according to their polarity. Some naturally occurring oils and fats are examined for the presence of the classes of lipid considered. Standards from representative groups are taken.

Requirements:

1. Thin layer plate of silica gel G
2. Separation chambers
3. Solvent (petroleum ether: diethylether: glacial acetic acid; 80:20:1)
4. Hydrocarbons (n-hexadecane and n-octadecane)
5. Cholesterol esters (Cholesterol acetate, Cholesterol oleate, Cholesterol stearate)
6. Vitamin A ester (Vitamin A palmitate)
7. Triacylglycerols (glycerol trioleate, glycerol tripalmitate)
8. Free fatty acids (oleic acid, palmitic acid, stearic acid)
9. Sterols (cholesterol)
10. Naturally occurring oils (olive oil, cod liver oil)
11. 2',7'-dichlorofluorescein (2 g/L in 95 % v/v ethanol)
12. Sulphuric acid (50 % v/v)
13. Oven at 110°C
14. Ultraviolet lamp.

Method

1. Clean the glass plates with ethanol; pour aqueous slurry of the gel on to their surface 250 mm thick
2. Activate the plates by heating at 110°C for 1 hr and allow cooling
3. Spot out 20-50 ml of 1 % w/v solution of each lipid in the solvent and develop the chromatogram
4. Locate the lipids by spraying with the dichlorofluorescein solution and view the plates in UV (270 nm)
5. The lipids show up as green fluorescent spots against a dark background. Alternatively, the spots can be visualized by spraying the plates with sulphuric acid followed by heating in the oven for 10 minutes.

Ion-Exchange Chromatography

The basis of this form of chromatography is the attraction between oppositely charged particles. Ion-exchange may be defined as the reversible change of ions in the solution with ions electrostatically bound to some sort of insoluble support medium. Since, many biological materials like amino acids and proteins have ionizable groups and they may carry a net positive or negative charge, this feature is utilized here for their separation. The net charge exhibited by such compounds depends on their pKa and on the pH of the solution.

Ion-exchange chromatography occurs in five distinct steps:

a. Diffusion of the ion to the exchanger surface. This occurs very quickly in a homogenous solution.
b. Diffusion of the ion through the matrix structure of the exchanger to the exchanger site. This is dependent on the degree of cross-linkage of the exchanger and the concentration of the solution.
c. Exchange of ions at the exchanger site: This occurs in equilibrium process–in case of cation exchanger as:

$$RSO_3^- \text{-------} Na^+ + {}^+NH_3R' \rightleftharpoons RSO_3^- \text{-------} {}^+NH_3R' + Na^+$$

Exchanger Ion	counter to be exchanged	charged molecule molecular ion	bound exchanged ion

d. Diffusion of the exchanged ion through the exchanger on the surface.
e. Selective desorption by the elutant and diffusion of the molecule into the external solution. The selective desorption of the bound molecule is achieved by change in pH and/ or ionic strength or by affinity elution.

The exchanger An ion exchanger is a solid that has chemically bound charged group to which ions are electrostatically bound; it can exchange these ions for ions in aqueous solution. There are two basic types of ionic exchangers on the basis of the ions they can exchange:

i. *Cation exchanger:* They possess negatively charged groups and attract positively charged molecules.
ii. *Anion exchanger:* They have a positively charged group which attracts negatively charged molecules, e.g. DEAE-cellulose, PAB-cellulose.

Basically three major groups of material are used in the construction of ion exchangers—polystyrene or polyphenolic resins; various types of cellulose and polymers of acrylamide and dextran.

Total exchange capacity Number of milliequivalents of exchangeable ions available, either per gram of dried exchanger or per unit volume of hydrated resin.

Buffers

- *Buffer rule* cationic buffers are used with anionic exchangers and anionic buffers are used with cationic exchangers. Buffers usually have counter ions in high ionic strength.

Experiment

Fractionation of normal rabbit serum proteins (IgG, IgA, IgM, macroglobulins and lipoproteins) using ion-exchange chromatography with DEAE-Sephadex A-50 column.

Requirements:

1. DEAE-Sephadex A-50 column
2. Phosphate buffer pH 8.0, 0.01 M, 0.08 M and 0.2 M
3. Normal rabbit serum

Method:

1. A column of DEAE-sephadex A-50 is packed
2. The column is equilibrated with 0.01 M phosphate buffer
3. Flow rate is adjusted to 2 ml/ 5 min.
4. 1 ml of normal rabbit serum dialyzed against 0.01 M phosphate buffer is loaded onto the column.
5. Fractions of 2 ml each are collected with 0.01 M phosphate buffer and OD_{280} noted for each fraction.
6. When OD is near zero, buffer is changed to 0.08 M phosphate buffer.
7. Fractions of 2 ml each are collected with 0.08 M phosphate buffer and OD_{280} noted for each fraction.
8. When OD is near zero, again, buffer is changed to 0.2 M phosphate buffer.
9. Same procedure repeated.
10. When OD came down to nearly zero, the column is washed with 0.01 M phosphate buffer + 0.05% NaCl w/v.
11. Later resin is swelled back with 0.01 M phosphate buffer.

Partition Chromatography

The separation of compounds that are readily soluble in organic liquids, but sparingly soluble in water, is carried out by adsorption chromatography, while ionizable water soluble compounds are best separated by ion exchange chromatography. Partition chromatography is intermediate between these two, and compounds that are soluble in both water and organic solvents are separated by partition methods.

When a compound is shaken with two immiscible solvents it will distribute itself unevenly between the two phases. Partition coefficient (α) is the ratio of the concentration of the compound in the two solvents.

$$\alpha = \frac{\text{Concentration of} \times \text{in solvent 1}}{\text{Concentration of} \times \text{in solvent 2}}$$

One solvent, usually water, is held on the stationary supporting phase, a column or a film of inert material. The other solvent forms the mobile phase that flows past the stationary phase. The components of a mixture are separated if their partition coefficients are sufficiently different.

Affinity Chromatography

Affinity chromatography exploits the unique property of extremely specific biological interactions to achieve separation and purification. It makes use of specific affinity between the substance to be isolated and a molecule that it can specifically bind (a ligand). Thus, in theory affinity chromatography is capable of giving absolute purification, even from a complex mixture, in a single step. In principle, these methods can be used to purify almost any macromolecule including enzymes, antibodies, specific and general classes of nucleic acids, vitamin binding proteins, repressors and other control elements.

The technique requires that the material to be isolated is capable of reversibly binding to a specific ligand, attached to an insoluble matrix.

$$\underset{\text{Matrix}}{\text{M}} \quad + \quad \underset{\substack{\text{Ligand} \\ \text{attached to matrix}}}{\text{L}} \rightleftharpoons \underset{\text{Complex}}{\text{ML}}$$

Affinity matrix. The ligand is covalently attached to a supporting medium so that the chromatographic material can be designed for a specific purification task. The matrix has to allow large molecules access to the binding sites and needs to have good flow properties. There should be no sites for nonspecific adsorption but must contain the functional groups to which ligands can be attached. A spacer arm is inserted between the matrix and the ligand so that large molecules can gain access to the binding sites. Spacer arm of 2-10°C atoms is optimal since a very short spacer arm can provide steric hindrance, while a long spacer arm increases the chances of nonspecific adsorption, especially of hydrophobic compounds.

Experiment

Elution of IgG fraction of normal rabbit serum using Protein-A affinity column.

Protein-A agarose column: Protein-A is derived from the cell wall of the bacterium *Staphylococcus aureus.* It has a high affinity for the Fc region of immunoglobulin gamma (IgG) and can be used for their isolation.

Requirements:

1. Protein-A sepharose column
2. Normal rabbit serum
3. 0.15 M phosphate buffer saline (PBS) pH 7.2-7.4
4. Glycine/HCl buffer 0.1 M pH 2.8.

Protocol:

1. Protein-A sepharose column is caliberated with PBS and its flow adjusted to 30 ml/hour.
2. 200 ml of normal rabbit serum loaded onto the column.
3. Each fraction of 1 ml collected with wash buffer PBS.
4. Absorbance 280 nm is taken for each fraction.
5. Once absorbance falls to near zero, buffer was changed to elution buffer glycine/HCl pH 2.8.
6. Fractions of 1 ml collected.
7. Absorbance 280 nm taken.
8. Plot graph of absorbance 280 nm against fraction numbers.
9. Column washed and re-equilibrated with PBS.

High Performance (Pressure) Liquid Chromatography (HPLC)

It is the most powerful, popular and versatile form of chromatography. The use of very fine particles with high pressure to maintain an adequate flow rate is HPLC. This method utilizes the principles of adsorption, partition, ion-exchange, exclusion and affinity that results in faster and better resolution of the separation.The resolving power of a column increases with the length of the column and the number of equilibrations per unit length of the column. The number of equilibrations is related to the surface area of the stationery phase. The flow rate of the column drops as the particle size decreases though the number of equilibrations is more. This problem is avoided by establishing a pressure difference across the top and bottom of the column to force the liquid (through pumps) into the bed.

10

Immunological Techniques

Antibodies are molecules which are generated by the body in response to a foriegn moiety called as antigen. Physiologically, presence of antibodies in blood is an indirect evidence of presence or encounter with an antigen. Thus, studies of antibodies in a system is an important parameter of analyzing the well being of one's body.

Simple antigen-antibody reactions *in vitro* can be detected by immunodiffusion (ID) techniques. These techniques are extremely specific and can detect and quantify specific molecular entities even in the presence of contaminating molecules. The ID techniques are essentially precipitation reactions in gels. When molecules such as soluble antigens diffuse from a homogenous solution into an agar gel containing a given concentration of antibody, the concentration of the antigen falls from a maximum at the solution-gel interface to zero at the leading edge of the region penetrated. Along this concentration gradient, at a point where the antigen concentration gives equivalence with a given concentration of antibody; a precipitate is formed. This region is called as zone of equivalence. This fact has been used since 1905 and later it developed into a range of highly sophisticated techniques. The following types of precipitation tests are in common use.

Single (Simple) Immunodiffusion

Oudin Tube Technique (One-dimensional)

This is a qualitative technique in which a solution or gel containing antigen(s) is layered onto a layer of agar containing antisera in a tube. As the antigen diffuses into the agar gel-containing antibody, the antigen-antibody complexes form a precipitate in the region where antigen and antibody concentration is equivalent.

Applications: To detect the presence of an antigen(s) in sera, culture filtrates, tissue extracts or fractions from gradient centrifugation.

Mancini's Radial ID Technique

In radial immunodiffusion to measure serum immunoglobulin concentrations, an agar gel is impregnated with an antiglobulin specific for one class (or subclass) of immunoglobulin for the species of interest, such that the concentration of the antiglobulin is constant throughout. The serum sample is placed in a well cut into the agar, then incubated to allow time for its diffusion. At the zone of optimal proportions of Ag (serum immunoglobulin) and Ab (antiglobulin), a precipitate will form in a ring around the gel. Since the concentration of the antiglobulin is constant, the diameter of the ring is proportional to the concentration of the Ag (serum immunoglobulin).

Standards, with known concentrations of immunoglobulin, are used to establish a standard curve. The diameter of the rings is measured and plotted for the standards on semi-log graph paper: ring diameter (in mm.) vs immunoglobulin concentration (in mg/dl on a log scale). A regression line is drawn through the points plotted for the standards. Then the concentration of the unknown sample is determined using its diameter and the standard curve (serum immunoglobulin) (Fig. 10.1).

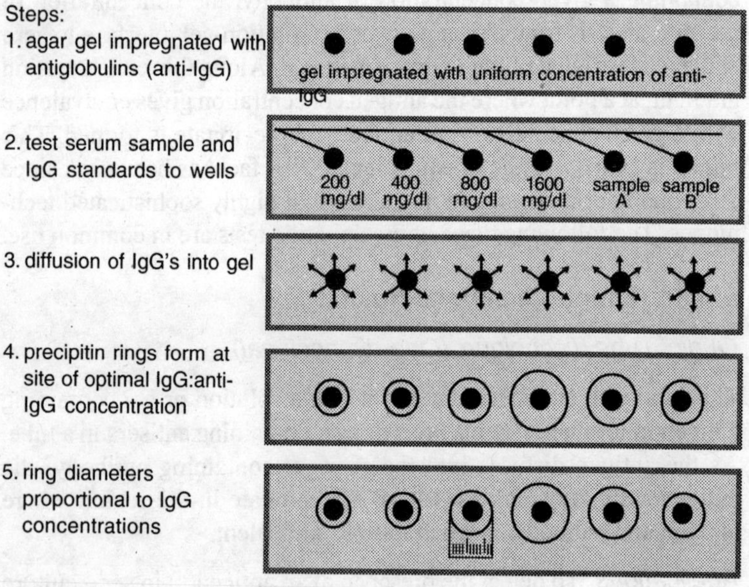

Fig. 10.1: Radial immunodiffusion

Applications. Routinely used for estimating the concentration of various immunoglobulins such as IgG and IgM in agammaglobulinemia and multiple myeloma respectively. Also used to determine the concentration of transferrin and alpha-fetoprotein (associated with certain liver tumors). One drawback to single radial immunodiffusion is the requirement of incubation overnight before reading the results.

Double Diffusion Techniques

Tube Assay

Similar to the Oudin method except that a layer of agar is placed between the antigens and antibodies, both reagents are allowed to diffuse towards each other, forming precipitation lines or equivalence points in the agar layer (Fig. 10.2).

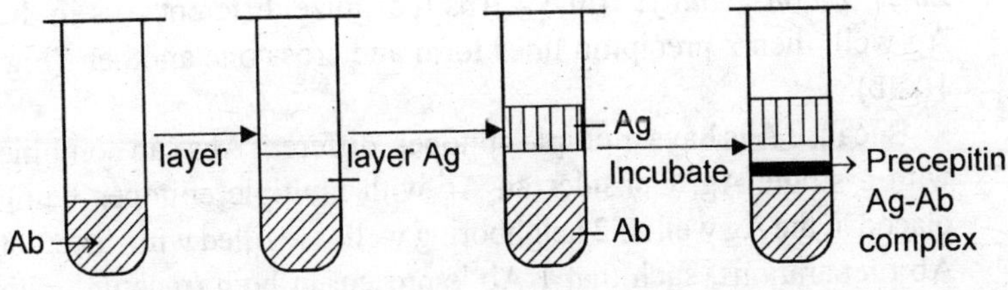

Fig. 10.2: Tube assay for double immunodiffusion

Ouchterlony Technique

The basic principle of agar gel immunodiffusion (AGID) is the formation of large Ag:Ab complexes that precipitate out of solution. This technique basically involve two stages:

Stage 1: Combine Ag and Ab; allow them to bind:

i. Add Ag to one well cut into an agar gel.
ii. Add source of Ab to a second well.
iii. Allow time for Ag and Ab to diffuse into the agar gel and combine.

Stage 2: Detect Ag:Ab binding:

i. At a point where there is approximately equimolar ratios of Ag and Ab, large complexes form and precipitate in the gel.
ii. The presence of a precipitin line indicates a positive test.

The lines formed by the Ag: Ab precipitates are called *precipitin* lines. Antibodies that react in this assay are called *precipitins.* The precipitation line is a hyperbola with its concavity towards the slower diffusing substance (usually antibody).

Qualitative Aspects of the Ouchterlony Technique

A modification (by Ouchterlony) of the technique places multiple wells at angles to one another. If different sources of Ab are placed in 2 wells, with a third well containing an Ag, it is possible to determine not only whether Abs are present, but whether they recognize the identical Ag.

- *Lines of identity:* If the 2 Abs do recognize the same Ag, a single precipitin line forms, creating a continuous arc between the 2 wells of Ab (Fig. 10.3a).
- *Lines of non-identity:* If the 2 Abs recognize different Ags in the Ag well, then 2 precipitin lines form and cross one another (Fig. 10.3b).

  Because Ags have multiple epitopes, different Abs can combine with a single Ag. Consider an Ag with multiple epitopes being placed in the Ag well. If 2 neighboring wells are filled with different Ab preparations, such that 1 Ab is present in both (reacting with one epitope) and another Ab is present in only one well, then two Ag:Ab reactions occur, and they share one reactant (the Ag).
- *Lines of partial identity:* A line of identity forms for the reaction in common between the 2 wells (the shared Ab). A line of non-identity also forms next to the well with the extra Ab, and overlaps the line

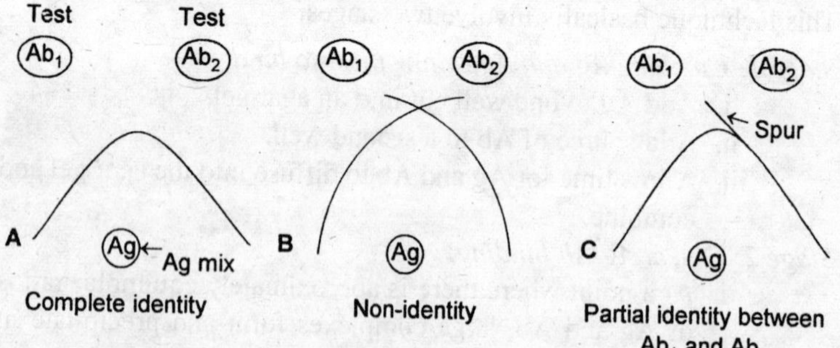

Fig. 10.3: Types of precipitin lines in ouchter long's technique

of identity. The resulting pattern appears as a line of identity with a "spur" and is called a "line of partial identity" (Fig. 10.3c).

The relative position of precipitin line yields a semiquantitative estimate of antigen concentration, i.e. more is the concentration of the antigen in solution, the farther from the antigen well will be the formation of the precipitation line (Fig. 10.3).

Immunoelectrophoretic Techniques

Immunoelectrophoresis

Immunoelectrophoresis combines two techniques to identify Ags in a sample:

- electrophoresis and
- immunodiffusion

Electrophoresis is a method of separating proteins in a sample (e.g., Ag) according to their net charge. The sample is applied to a gel, the gel is placed in an electrolyte solution, and a current is applied to the electrolyte solution. Positively charged proteins, such as many Abs, migrate through the gel toward the cathode (negative terminal). Negatively charged proteins, such as albumin, migrate through the gel toward the anode (positive terminal), depending on the net charge of the protein.

In immunoelectrophoresis, a gel is prepared and a well is slots cut into it. The Ag mixture (usually a serum sample) is placed in the well and electrophoresis is performed to separate the proteins in the sample. Then an Ab (or mixture of Abs) is added to the slots in the gel. The separated Ags and the Abs migrate toward one another and form precipitin arcs at the region of optimal concentrations (Fig. 10.4).

Immunoelectrophoresis is not often used anymore. Usually, it is performed to detect immunoglobulin classes or complement proteins in plasma. Immunodeficiencies or excesses of immunoglobulin classes can be detected with this technique.

Applications. Identification of a specific antigen when other antigens are also present. In clinical immunology, semiquantitative information regarding immunoglobulin concentration and identification of myeloma proteins.

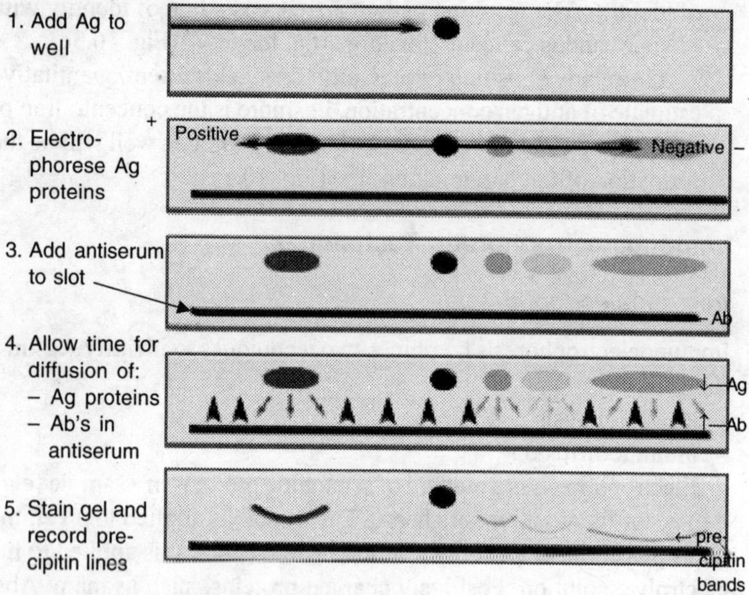

Fig. 10.4: Immunoelectrophoresis

Counter Current Immunoelectrophoresis (Cross Over Electrophoresis)

This technique takes advantages of cathodal migration of gamma-globulins. A voltage is applied to Ag, which migrates towards positive pole in agar. Hence, precipitation lines are formed more rapidly than the Ouchterlony method. This method is more sensitive as all the molecules migrate towards each other rather than diffusing radially.

Applications. This technique is especially useful in forensic medicine. It is used for detection of hepatitis B Ag, Anti-HBV antibodies and Anti-DNA antibodies. As many as 12 samples may be tested on one agar covered microscope slide.

Rocket Electrophoresis (Quantitative Method)

This technique is similar to the single radial ID technique (Mancini's). The antigen sample is loaded into wells, cut in agar containing specific antisera. On applying direct electric current most antigens migrate towards the anode. The precipitation line formed at equivalence is in the manner of rocket proportional to the antigen concentration. A plot of rocket height against concentration will be linear. By the use of standards and calibration curve, the concentration of antigen solution may be determined. It is suitable for proteins such as albumin, transferrin, and ceruloplasmin (Fig. 10.5).

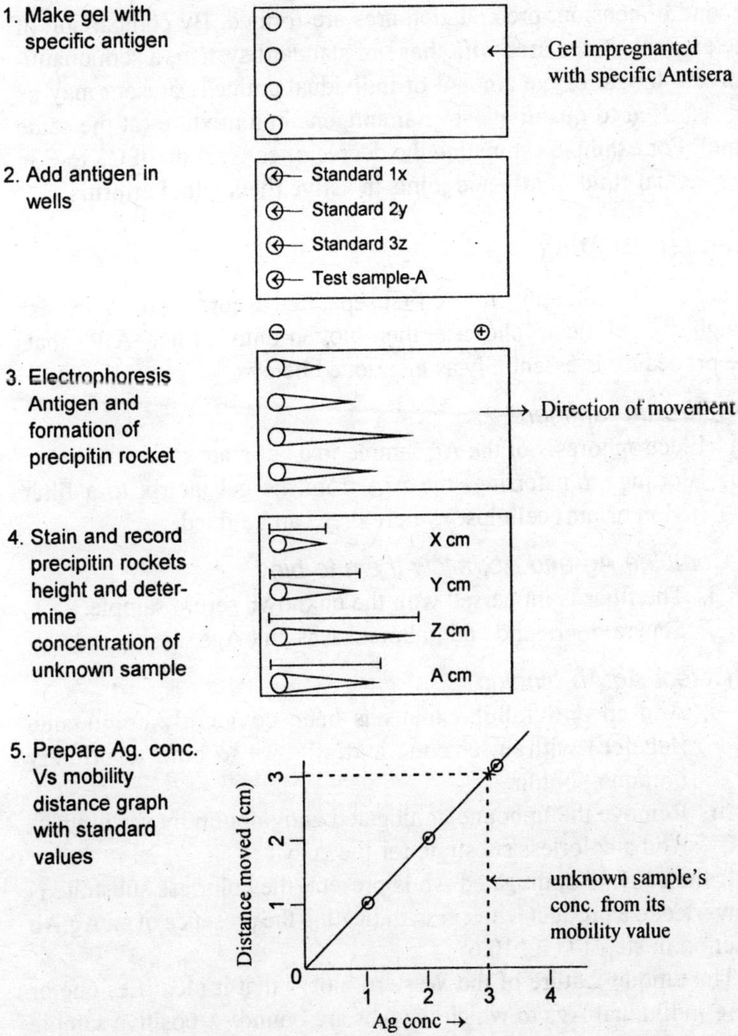

Fig. 10.5: Rocket electrophoresis (Mancini's technique)

Laurell's Two-dimensional Electrophoresis

This technique combines electrophoretic separation in a molecular sieving medium with the specificity and speed of rocket electrophoresis. Initially antigens are separated by agar electrophoresis in one dimension. The slice of gel is transferred into a square glass plate containing suitable antisera in a layer of agar. After rocket IE in the second dimension, precipitation arcs are formed. By comparison of the area under the arcs with those of standard system, a semiquantitative estimate of the amount of individual antigens present may be made. Used to quantitate several antigens in a mixture (at the same time). For example estimating the degree of conversion of C3 to C3c in synovial fluid of affected joints in active rheumatoid arthritis.

Western Blotting

In a western blot, antigens are first separated according to molecular weight by gel electrophoresis, then blotted onto a filter. After that, the procedure is essentially as mentioned below:

Prepare the antigen

i. Electrophoresis of the Ag sample in a gel matrix.
ii. Blotting (transferring) the Ags from the gel matrix to a filter (nylon or nitrocellulose) where they can be fixed.

1. *Combine Ag and Ab; allow them to bind*
   i. The filter is immersed with the unknown serum sample.
   ii. Separating bound and unbound Abs and Ags.
2. *Detect Ag:Ab binding*
   i. Add an antiglobulin that has been covalently conjugated (labeled) with an enzyme and allow it to bind to primary immunoglobulin.
   ii. Remove the unbound conjugated antiglobulin by washing.
   iii. Add a colorless substrate for the enzyme.

If the enzyme-conjugated Ab is present, the colorless substrate is converted to a product with color, indicating the presence of an Ag:Ab reaction in step 1 (Fig. 10.6).

The unique feature of the Western blot is that it identifies one or more individual Ags to which the Abs are bound. A positive sample will show binding of the enzyme-labeled antiglobulin at the particular

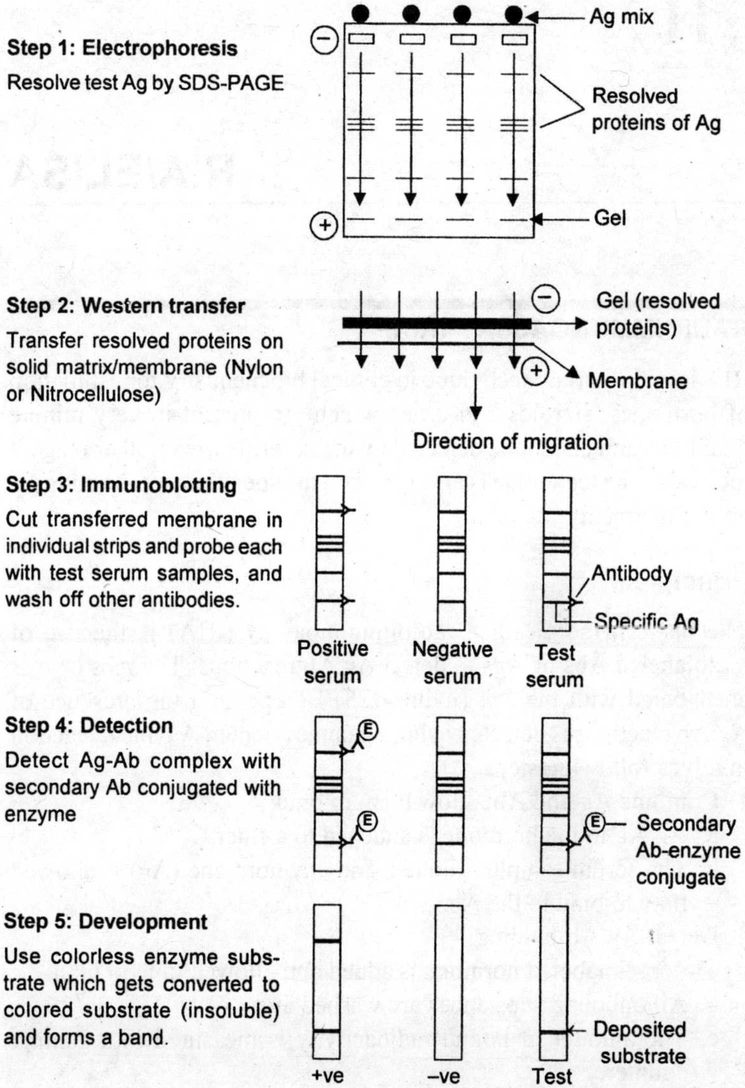

Fig. 10.6: Western transfer and immunoblotting

sites where Ags of the infectious agent are known to migrate in electrophoresis. If there is binding at other sites, the sample is considered negative because the binding is to a contaminating Ag in the preparation.

11

RIA/ELISA

RADIOIMMUNOASSAY (RIA)

RIA is an important technique in clinical biochemistry for estimation of hormones, steroids and drugs which are present in very minute quantities and cannot be detected by the colorimetric or other reagent methods. The technique is also based on the specificity of the antigen-antibody reaction.

Principle

The basic principle of a radioimmunoassay (RIA) is the use of radiolabeled Abs or Ags to detect Ag:Ab reactions. The Abs or Ags are labeled with the ^{125}I (iodine-125) isotope, and the presence of Ag:Ab reactions is detected using a gamma counter. A typical reaction involves following steps.

1. Combine Ag and Ab; allow them to bind:
   a. An Ab to the hormone is attached to a filter
   b. The serum sample is added, and any hormone (Ag) is allowed time to bind to the Ab.
2. Detect Ag:Ab binding:
   a. A radiolabeled hormone is added and allowed time to bind.
   b. All unbound substances are washed away.
   c. The amount of bound radioactivity is measured in a gamma counter.

The presence of the hormone in the serum sample inhibits binding of the radiolabeled hormone. Thus, the amount of radioactivity present in the test is inversely proportional to the amount of hormone in the serum sample. A standard curve using increasing amounts of known concentrations of the hormone is used to determine the quantity in the sample.

Requirements

Apart from the test samples (unlabeled Ag of unknown concentrations), e.g. blood, serum, urine, etc. the following are required.

1. *Labeled antigen (Tracer):* The pure antigen tagged with a radioisotope. Usually the tyrosine in protein antigen is labeled with I^{125} either by chloramine T or by lactoperoxidase method. Non-protein antigens are labeled with tritium.
2. *Antibody* against the test substance should be available with high specificity, high titer and high affinity.
3. *Standard antigen* (unlabeled Ag of known conc.) must be available in pure form.
4. A suitable buffer of pH 7-9.
5. *Scintillation counter*
   a. Gamma counter for I^{125} labeled antigen with high sensitivity and low half-life.
   b. Beta counter for H^3 labeled antigen with lower sensitivity but higher half-life.

Methodology

1. A series of immuno tubes are taken in which varying amounts of pure antigen are incubated with fixed amounts of the labeled antigen and immobilized antibody for 6 hours.
2. The free and the bound antigens are separated and the radioactivity is counted in the bound Ag*Ab fraction.
3. The test sample with the unknown amount of antigen is processed similarly.
4. Known quantity of unlabeled Ag as different dilutions of standards are taken to draw a standard curve (dose response curve).
5. By referring to the standard curve, the amount of antigen can be obtained.

Methods of Separation of Bound and Unbound Antigen

1. Ion-exchange chromatography.
2. Adsorption of free antigen on charcoal followed by centrifugation leaving the bound Ag*– Ab in the supernatant.
3. Using second antibody against the first antibody.

4. Salt precipitation of Ag* Ab complex.
5. Immobilization of the antibody on a solid support and washing away of the free antigen.
6. Using Protein-A of *Staphylococcus aureus*. This has high affinity for human lgG (Fig 11.1).

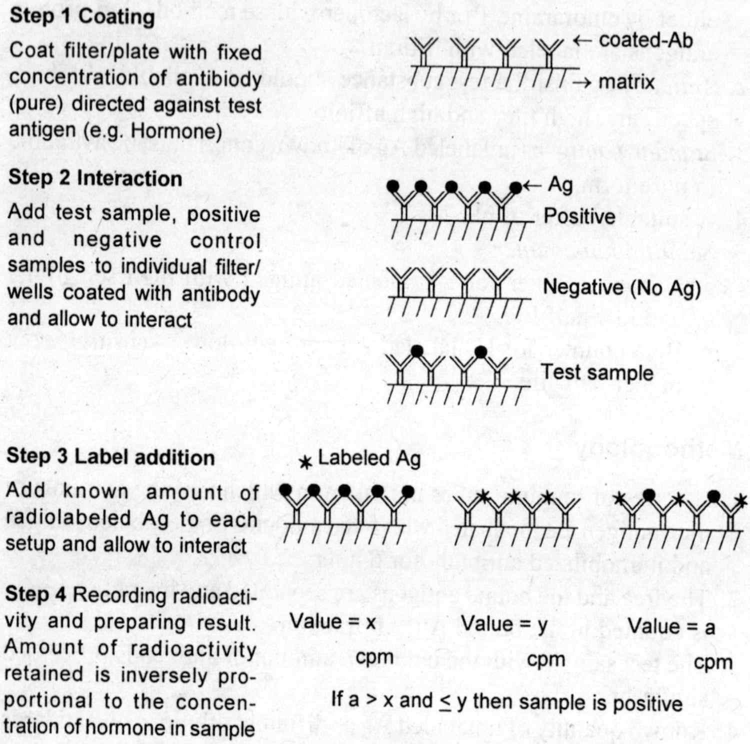

Fig. 11.1: Principle of RIA

Advantages of RIA

1. It can be used to assay any compound which is immunogenic, available in pure form and can be radiolabeled.
2. It is a very sensitive test.
3. It is highly specific and reproducible.
4. It has a broad range of measurement.
5. It can be automated.

Disadvantages of RIA

1. Very high cost of equipments and reagents.
2. Half life of I^{125} is 60 days which requires frequent ordering.
3. Hazards of radioactivity.
4. Lengthy procedure.

Applications

Used in the measurement of peptide/steroid hormones such as T3, T4, TSH, hCG progesterone, etc. in clinical chemistry. RIAs are highly sensitive and quantitative, capable of detecting small amounts of Ag or Ab. As a result, they are often used to measure the quantities of hormones or drugs present in a patient's serum. Often, RIAs are performed in solution, rather than on filters. Ag:Ab complexes precipitate from solution, and the amount of radioactivity in the supernatant is measured. In this case, the amount of radioactivity present in the supernatant, representing unbound radiolabeled hormone, is proportional to the directly proportional to the amount of hormone in the sample.

Another use of the RIA is to measure the quantities of serum IgE antibodies specific for various allergens in a patient's serum, in which case it is called a Radio Allergo Sorbent Test (RAST). In this case, the test is performed similar to an ELISA for Ab, using radiolabeled antiglobulins specific for IgE, rather enzyme-labeled antiglobulins. However, this test has been almost completely replaced by ELISAs.

ENZYME-LINKED IMMUNOSORBENT ASSAY (ELISA)

An ELISA can be used to detect either the presence of Abs or Ags in a sample, depending on how the test is designed.

Principle

It is similar in principle to RIA. The basic principle of an ELISA is to use an immunoglobulin-coupled enzyme to detect the binding of Ag and Ab. The enzyme converts a colorless substrate (chromogen) to a colored product, indicating the presence of Ag:Ab binding. The detection depends on spectrophotometric assays.

Methodology

To Detect Ags in a sample:

1. Combine Ag and Ab; allow them to bind:
   i. An Ab that reacts with the Ag is firmly attached to a surface
   ii. Sample being tested (containing Ag) is added, allowed to incubate
2. Detect Ag:Ab binding:
   i. A second Ab that reacts with the primary Ab and that is covalently attached to an enzyme (i.e., enzyme-linked) is added allowed to incubate, then unbound enzyme-linked Abs are washed from the surface
   ii. A colorless substrate of the enzyme is added
   iii. If the enzyme-linked Ab bound to Ags on the surface, the enzyme will convert the colorless substrate to a colored product, which is detected spectrophotometrically.

To Detect Abs in a Sample—Methodology

1. The Ag is adsorbed onto a solid support which may be cellulose, paper or plastic.
2. The unbound Ag is then washed away and the adsorbent is blocked with excess of an irrelevant protein to prevent any subsequent non-specific binding of proteins.
3. The specific antibody is then added. The antibody binds very specifically and with high affinity to the antigen.
4. This bound antibody is then detected by ligand. The ligand is usually another Ab (2nd antibody) directed against the first antibody.
5. These ligands are linked to enzymes. The enzymes should be stable at room temperature, should have high turnover number, be cheap and easily available, with products that are chromogenic and with no cross-reactivity. The most commonly used enzymes are horse radish peroxidase or alkaline phosphatase. The unbound ligand is washed away.
6. The bound ligand is visualized by addition of a chromogen, a colorless substance which is converted into a colored complex by the enzyme bound to the ligand. This colored end product is assayed spectrophotometrically.

Some clinically important substances commonly measured by ELISA include.

Antigens

1. Alfa-fetoprotein
2. *Human chorionic gonadotropin (hCG)* The hCG levels in the serum and urine begin to rise soon after the onset of pregnancy. It also rises due to trophoblastic tumors. The conventional test of latex agglutination takes a long time to become positive. ELISA is more sensitive for detection of pregnancy and can detect urinary hCG within 15 days of conception. The test urine is coated on the plate and the nonspecific binding is blocked with bovine serum albumin. The plate is then washed with phosphate buffered saline and anti-hCG antibody is added. The bound antibody is then detected by antibody coupled to horse radish peroxidase. The substrate o-phenylene diamine (OPD) and nascent oxygen, released from H_2O_2 by the action of the enzyme peroxidase, react to form a brown colored complex. The absorbance is read at 490 nm.
3. Hepatitis B
4. IgG
5. HIV.

Antibodies

1. Anti-DNA antibodies
2. Anti-rubella antibodies
3. Anti-*Toxoplasma gonodii* antibodies

Types of ELISA

Different types of ELISA have been developed depending on qualitative detection and quantitative measurement.

1. *Direct ELISA.* Antigen is coated on the plates. Enzyme is conjugated with the primary antibody. Ag is detected here.

2. *Indirect ELISA.* Antigen is coated on the plates. Enzyme is conjugated with the secondary antibody. Ab is detected here.

3. *Sandwich ELISA.* Antigen is sandwiched between two primary antibodies recognizing two different epitopes of the antigen. First antibody is coated on the plates. Second antibody, which is added after the antigen addition, is linked to the enzyme. It is an Ag detection test.

4. *Competitive ELISA* Similar to RIA. Both unknown antigen (sample) and the known antigen (standard) compete with each other for a fixed amount of antibody. Ag is detected (Fig. 11.2).

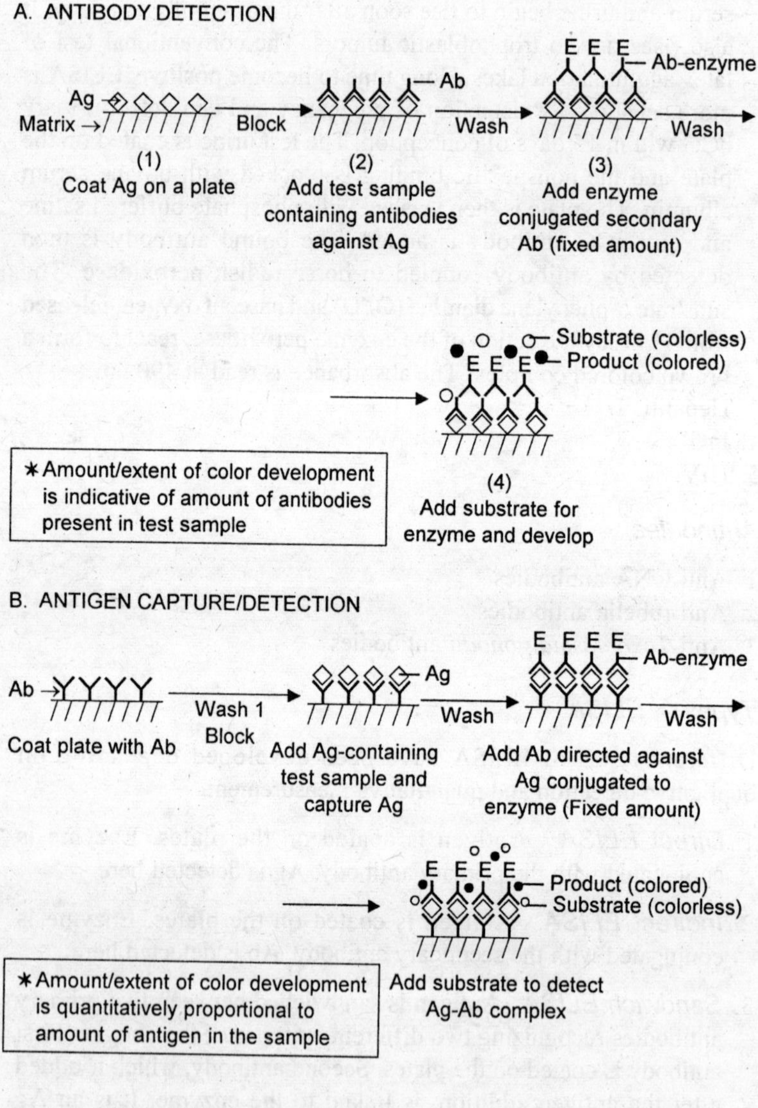

Fig. 11.2: Representation of an ELISA to detect antibodies specific to Ag

Example

The competitive ELISA can detect Abs in a sample. It is based on the principle that Abs in the sample will bind to an Ag and then inhibit binding of an enzyme-linked Ab that reacts with the Ag (i.e., competes for binding).

1. Combine Ag and Ab; allow them to bind:
   i. The Ag is firmly attached to a surface (usually a plastic well or filter)
   ii. Sample being tested is added and allowed to incubate
2. Detect Ag:Ab binding:
   i. An enzyme-linked Ab that reacts with the Ag is added, allowed to incubate, and then washed from the surface
   ii. A colorless substrate of the enzyme is added
   iii. If the sample contained Abs that react with the Ag, they would inhibit binding of the enzyme-labeled Ab and no color reaction would occur.
   iv. If the sample does not contain Abs that react with the Ag, the enzyme-labeled Ab would bind and a color reaction would occur.

Note: In the competitive ELISA, no color reaction is a POSITIVE result, and a color reaction is a NEGATIVE result.

12

General Molecular Biology Techniques—Principles and Processes

"All science is surreal, but the proofs are for real"

Molecular biology as a discipline involves studying biology at molecular level. The molecules which need to be studied to understand various processes broadly come in three categories *viz.* DNA, RNA and proteins. By the rule book of molecular biology, the central dogma is centered on these three entities in a largely linear process,

$$\text{DNA} \leftarrow \text{DNA} \leftrightarrows \text{RNA} \rightarrow \text{Protein}$$

This flow of information is very generalized and other modifications of this flow are known in the biological kingdom. Since, they are outside the scope of this book they are not discussed herein. The simple relationship of the participating molecules is discussed below.

a. *DNA*–**D**eoxyribose **N**ucleic **A**cid, genetic material, encodes the genetic information which govern not only the hereditary information but also all the normal processes of an organism. The process of DNA that governs its own copying is called as replication.

b. *RNA*–**R**ibose **N**ucleic **A**cid, messenger of DNA, carries the information of the cellular processes from the DNA. The process which leads to synthesis of RNA from a DNA template is called as transcription.

c. *Protein*–building blocks of a body. Governs 'all' the processes in a living organism. The process of protein synthesis from basic amino acids from information present on messenger RNA is termed as translation.

It is established that a good knowledge of biochemistry is essential before an understanding of molecular biology can be made. This is basically because

Molecular biology = genetics + biochemistry

The application of molecular biology or recombinant DNA technology in the analysis of disease has expanded greatly since its introduction in around 1978, when it was first reported that thalassemia syndromes result from the unbalanced synthesis of the globin genes, which became the first genetic disorder to be described in detail at the molecular level. At the clinical level, the new genetic methods have had their greatest impact on diagnosis and that's what we would address here. Development of procedures which facilitated detection of specific 'gene defects' or mutations related to a disease process, their distribution and frequency of occurrence in a population, in detection of carrier in case of familial inheritance disorders and in prenatal diagnosis have helped medicine in a unparallel manner. With a catalog of clinically relevant gene mutations for which individuals may be surveyed, these procedures can be applied with great precision and effect.

Basic Experiments in Molecular Biology

Since the field of molecular biology revolves essentially around three components–DNA, RNA and proteins, many experiments can be planned and performed on these three 'subjects' to understand how the rest of molecular biology rests on them. The experiment in this section would essentially involve isolation of DNA, RNA and proteins and their subsequent analysis by various biochemical techniques like spectrophotometry, electrophoresis, chromatography, etc.

Isolation and biochemical analysis procedures:

1. Genomic DNA isolation, spectrophotometric evaluation, gene amplification by PCR, karyotyping, fluorescence *in situ* hybridization (FISH)
2. RNA isolation, spectrophotometric evaluation,
3. Protein isolation, specific protein analysis by western blotting.

DNA TECHNIQUES

Genomic DNA Isolation

The entire genetic material of an organism is called a genome. Isolation of the intact genomic DNA from both microorganisms and higher multicellular organisms does not need some special setup and can be performed in a routine laboratory setup. Isolation of DNA is the basic requirement of any DNA–based diagnosis techniques like PCR of infectious agent or genetic analysis of any inherited disorder.

Prior to the isolation of DNA, it is necessary to know what type of cells or tissue should be used for DNA isolation, as some types of cells have high DNase activity and DNA isolated from such cells is of poor quality because of degradation during isolation. Certain types of cells have low DNA to cell mass ratio hence yield low amounts. From this point of view thymus is the best source followed by lymphoid cells and spleen.

Requirements

1. Lysis buffer–50 mM Tris.HCl, pH 8.0; 10 mM EDTA; 100 mM NaCl and 200 μg/ml RNase A.
2. SDS–20%
3. Proteinase K–20 mg/ml in deionized water
4. Tris buffered phenol, pH 8.0
5. Saturated chloroform: Isoamyl alcohol (24:1 mix of chloroform: isoamyl alcohol)
7. Ethanol (kept at-20°C)
8. TE buffer (10 mM Tris.HCl, pH 8.0; 1 mM EDTA in sterile deionized water)

Methodology and Principle

1. Take a small amount of cells (grown *in vitro*) or tissue section and weight them. Resuspend the cells in lysis buffer (1 ml per 100 mg weight) and homogenize thoroughly [homogenization can be performed by repetitive pipetting or passing the suspension through a 22/23 G needle].

DNA is rapidly degraded and care should be taken to avoid stresses on it, mechanical stress and extreme physical or chemical conditions should be avoided.

2. Add SDS to 2% and proteinase K to 100 μg/ml (final concentrations) to the suspension.

   Presence of SDS ruptures the cells and liberates the proteins and nucleic acid including DNA/RNA in the supernatant. Proteinase K denatures the proteins, since it is not inhibited by the presence of SDS, this protease can be used in conjunction.
3. Incubate the mix at 55°C for 2–3 hours. Check the lysate at this stage, it should be viscous and if it is not then add another 100 μg/ml of proteinase K and incubate mix at 55°C for 2 hours.
4. Add equal volume of buffered phenol to the lysate, keep on rocker platform for 10 minutes with gentle shaking (any vigorous mixing at this and subsequent stages can lead to shearing of DNA).

   Phenol extraction removes all the proteins from the lysate, leaving behind DNA in the aqueous phase.
5. Centrifuge at 4°C for 15 minutes at 6000 rpm.
6. Isolate upper aqueous phase and add equal volume of saturated chloroform to it.

   Presence of even trace amounts of phenol in the DNA can interfere with subsequent applications of DNA like enzymatic digestion and PCR. To remove phenol completely, chloroform extractions are performed. Besides this application, chloroform is a potent deproteinising agent and also helps in removing the rest of protein from the DNA preparation.
7. Mix by gentle inversion and keep at rocker platform for 5 minutes at RT.
8. Centrifuge at 4°C for 15 minutes at 6000 rpm and collect the upper aqueous phase and repeat the chloroform extractions till aqueous phase is clear.
9. Add three volumes of chilled ethanol or 0.6 volumes of isopropanol and mix by inversion. Appearance of a wooly genomic DNA spool indicates isolation of pure genomic DNA.

   Addition of water-miscible organic solvents like ethanol or isopropanol which lower the dielectric constant of water leads to precipitation of DNA by salting out phenomenon. Presence of even very low amounts of salt at this stage (which comes from previous steps) is enough to precipitate the DNA.

10. Pellet the DNA by centrifugation at 12000 rpm at 4°C for 30 minutes.
11. Wash the pellet once with 70% ethanol (add 0.5 ml of 70% chilled ethanol, centrifuge at 12000 rpm for 10 minutes at 4°C).
    This step facilitates the removal of the traces of salt precipitated with DNA.
12. Discard supernatant and air dry the pellet at 37°C.
13. Resuspend the pellet in TE buffer (100 μl for 100 mg cells).
14. Estimate the purity and yield of DNA obtained by spectrophotometric analysis.

Spectrophotometric Analysis of Purity and Yield of DNA

The nucleic acids absorb strongly in the ultraviolet region of the spectrum due to conjugated double bond systems of the constituent purine and pyrimidines. They show characteristic absorption maxima at 260 nm. To estimate the purity and yield of DNA, the absorption of DNA sample is analyzed at 260 nm and 280 nm. A ratio of A_{260}/A_{280} gives a fairly good estimation about the purity of DNA. A ratio of 1.6–1.8 is considered sufficiently pure whereas a ratio of 2.0 indicates towards the presence of degradation byproducts of DNA and a ratio below 1.6 indicates towards the presence of contaminating protein in DNA sample.

The yield of DNA is calculated from the absorbance of a pure sample at 260 nm. For an absorbance of 1, the amount of double stranded DNA is around 50 μg, whereas it is around 33 μg for oligonucleotides (primers) and single stranded DNA and 40 μg for RNA.

Methodology

1. Dilute the isolated DNA in water in a dilution of 1: 50 and 1: 100, i.e. 20 μl DNA in 980 μl water and 10 μl in 990 μl.
2. Switch on the spectrophotometer and the UV lamp and let it warm for 15–20 mins.
3. Set the background to zero with 20 μl TE in 980 μl water in a quartz cuvette at 260 nm (it is important to note that only quartz cuvettes can be used in ultraviolet wavelength range, as glass cuvettes absorb at this wavelength).
4. Take the absorbance of the DNA samples at 260 nm.

5. Calculate the total absorbance of the sample by multiplying the absorbance of the diluted sample with the dilution factor, i.e. absorbance of 1 : 50 diluted sample × 50 or absorbance of 1 : 100 diluted sample × 100 would yield the net absorbance of the DNA sample. To calculate the total yields multiply the total absorbance by the volume of DNA sample (in ml). For example,

   DNA resuspension volume, V = 100 μl.
   Dilution factor, X = 1 : 50
   OD of the diluted product, A = 0.02.
   Absorbance of total sample, At = A × X = 0.02 × 50 = 1.
   Therefore, actual OD = At × V = 1 × 0.1 = 0.1.

   By the absorbance law,

   OD_{260} 1 = 50 μg DNA

   Therefore, OD_{260} 0.1 = 5 μg DNA.

Polymerase Chain Reaction (PCR)

PCR is the single technology which has revolutionized the current molecular biology more than any other technology. It is of an accepted understanding that without PCR we would not have reached the place where we are today. Be it DNA based diagnosis, elucidation of genomic information of various organisms, expression of foreign proteins in other hosts, elucidation of genetic or inborn errors, characterization of expression of genes in various disease conditions and many other research areas PCR has proved its potential in everything. Kary Mullis invented the polymerase chain reaction in 1984 and first clinical application of the techniques was in detection and identification of sickle cell mutation. And since the technique requires minute amount of sample, takes hours rather than days and can be effectively automated, PCR has rapidly found its way into most clinical and research laboratories.

Using PCR, we can selectively copy segments of DNA repeatedly to generate large quantities of the same for further analysis. For this, we need to know the DNA sequences flanking the region to be amplified. In this technique, a denatured DNA sample is incubated with DNA polymerase, precursor dNTPs and two oligonucleotides (primers) whose sequence flank the DNA sequence of interest so that they direct the DNA polymerase to synthesize new complimentary strands.

A generalized PCR reaction consisting of three stages: denaturation of the template DNA by heat, annealing of the oligonucleotide primers to the single-stranded target sequence(s), and extension of the annealed primers by a thermostable DNA polymerase to form the amplicon or the amplified segment. The use of a thermostable DNA polymerase such as Taq polymerase eliminates the need to add fresh enzyme after each heat denaturation step. Hence, in the presence of sufficient quantities of primers and dNTPs, the PCR is carried out simply by cyclically varying the temperatures. Twenty cycles of PCR can give a increase the amount of a target DNA by almost one million folds. The amplified DNA can be further analyzed by electrophoresis, southern hybridization, RFLP analysis or direct sequencing.

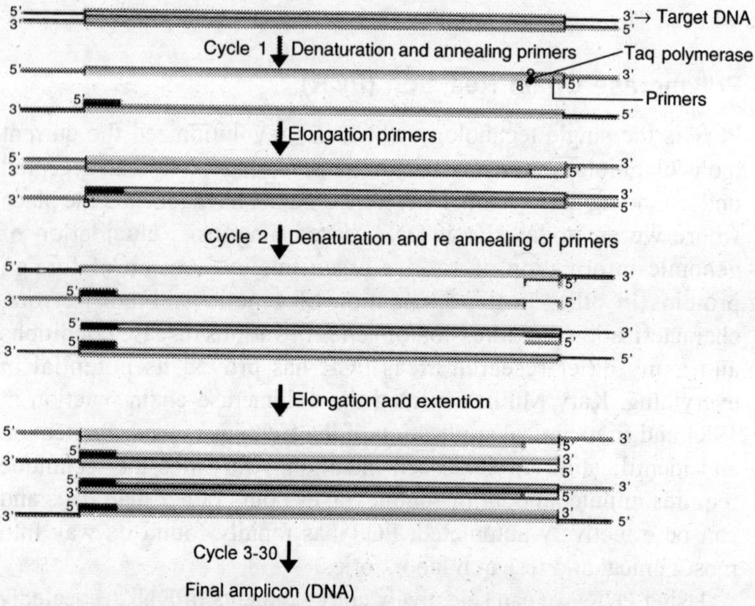

Fig. 12.1: Representation of amplification of a specific gene target using PCR

Amplification Factors

1. *Primers:* The most important factor regulating the amplification. The annealing temperature of the primer is defined as the temperature at which the primer can bind specifically to the target

DNA sequence. It should be low enough to allow primer DNA–target DNA hybrid formation along with being high enough to maintain stringency such that the primer DNA should not form weak hybrids with nonspecific regions allowing some mismatches. For this the annealing temperature should be as close as possible to the melting temperature of the primers (Tm-melting temperature is the temperature at which the primers would denature and fall off from the target DNA). The Tm of primers is calculated by the formula $4 \times (G+C) + 2 \times (A+T) \times n/20$ where A, G, C and T are the number of respective nucleotides in the primers and n is the nucleotide length of primer.

2. *Mg^{2+} ion concentration:* Important divalent ion required for activity of polymerase.
3. *Polymerase: Taq* DNA polymerase isolated from bacteria *Thermus aquaticus* is most commonly used enzyme. It has a high turnover, but lacks the proofreading capacity. For this activity many other enzymes have been isolated and are in use like *Pfu* DNA polymerase, *Vent* polymerase, T4 polymerase, etc. All these enzymes have a 3' exonuclease activity, which is desired for proof-reading activity. Because of this activity, the turnover or processing speed of these enzymes is less.

Applications

1. For diagnosis of rare genetic or pathological disorders.
2. For detection of nucleotide sequences of infectious agents for identification and diagnosis (e.g. viruses, bacteria).
3. In forensic science for analysis of samples as small as single hair roots, etc. to identify the donor.
4. In molecular paleontology to study the process of evolution and development
5. Cloning of PCR product for further study, like sequencing, expression, etc.

Variations of PCR

1. *RT-PCR:* In RT-PCR, the template DNA is prepared from mRNA using the enzyme reverse transcriptase, which uses RNA as template and synthesizes complimentary DNA also called as cDNA.

2. *Nested PCR:* This technique uses two sets of primers—one within the other to improve the fidelity of PCR.
3. *Multiplex PCR:* Multiple templates are amplified in the same reaction using different sets of primers.
4. *Quantitative PCR or real time PCR:* Uses an internal standard to quantify the amount of PCR amplified products almost at each cycle in real time. Hence, this type of PCR is also called as real-time PCR.
5. *Hot start PCR:* To avoid the nonspecific binding of primers leading to nonspecific amplification, the reaction is initiated by addition of one of the constituents (mostly the polymerase enzyme) in the cocktail only after the initial denaturation step is over.

Requirements

1. Template DNA
2. Specific gene primers (prepared at a concentration of 20 μM)
3. 10 mM dNTP mix (solution containing each of the dNTPs in a concentration of 10 mM)
4. DNA polymerase (*Taq* polymerase)
5. Amplification buffer
6. $MgCl_2$ or $MgSO_4$
7. Deionized water.

Methodology

1. Prepare a PCR cocktail of following ingredients in the mentioned order:

Component	*Stock concentration*	*Working concentration*
Amplification buffer	10X	1X
$MgCl_2$	25 mM	1.5–3.0 mM
Primers	20 μM	0.5 μM
dNTPs	10 mM	200 μM
Taq polymerase	5U/ μl	0.5 U/ reaction of 20 μl

H_2O to make up the volume to 20 μl (including the volume of template).

Keep the cocktail on ice.

2. Add template (25–250 ng of genomic DNA) to the cocktail tubes. For multiple reaction tubes, make common cocktail, then dispense it in individual tubes, followed by addition of template DNA.
3. Immediately after addition of template subject the tubes to PCR cycling, a generalized cycling program is given below:

Step	*Temperature*	*Duration*	
Initial denaturation	94°C	5–10 minutes	
Denaturation	94°C	30 seconds	30-35 cycles
Annealing of primers	5°C below Tm of primers	30 seconds	30-35 cycles
Extention of the amplified product	72°C	1 min per kb of DNA	30-35 cycles
Final extension	72°C	5-10 minutes.	

4. After the amplification, analyze the amplified products by agarose gel electrophoresis or by polyacrylamide gel electrophoresis.

Karyotyping

Recent advances in human genome mapping and the inheritance database have provided us with molecular tools to study a vast majority of inheritance related disorders. For disorders in which various biochemical, molecular and cytogenetic defects have been identified and characterized, prenatal diagnosis is possible and if the fetus is detected to have such a complication, selective termination or MTP is possible.

This process involves testing of fetal cells for genetic diagnosis. During the second trimester of pregnancy (15–16 weeks of gestation) fetal cells can be obtained by amniocentesis or by chorionic villus sampling in the first trimester (9–12 weeks gestation). It has also been suggested to perform such an analysis prior to implantation in the cases of *in vitro* fertilization and in such cases it is called as pre-implantation genetic diagnosis. Such an analysis allows genetically at risk couples to start off a family with a pregnancy of an unaffected fetus and avoid the need to consider selective termination later in the gestation.

A karyotype is technically "a photomicrograph of chromosomes arranged according to a standard classification". Karyotyping can also be mentioned as chromosome analysis. Karyotyping is a test to identify chromosome abnormalities as the cause of malformation or disease.

This test can, count the number of chromosomes, look for structural changes in chromosomes and the results may indicate genetic changes linked to a disease.

The test can be performed on a sample of blood, bone marrow, amniotic fluid, or placental tissue. The specimen is grown in tissue culture in the laboratory. Then, the cells are harvested, and the chromosomes are stained and viewed under the microscope. They are photographed to provide a karyotype, which shows the arrangement of the chromosomes. Certain abnormalities can be identified through the number or arrangement of the chromosomes.

Requirements

1. Phytohemagglutin (PHA) enriched RPMI-1640 media
2. Colcemid solution, 10 µg per ml, in Hanks balanced salt solution (HBSS)
3. Hypertonic KCl, 0.075 M
4. Fixative, 3 parts anhydrous methanol to 1 part glacial acetic acid (3:1)
5. Giemsa stock solution
6. Giemsa working solution 1% at pH 6.8
7. Phosphate buffer 0.025 M (3.4 g KH_2PO_4 per liter adjusted to pH 6.8 with KOH)
8. Trypsin (1:250), 1% solution in water
9. Methanol
10. Acridine orange.

Methodology

1. Autoclave heparinized tubes
2. Add 5 ml of PHA enriched RPMI-1640 Media to 15 ml culture tubes and freeze.
3. Add 3-4 drops of blood to each tube (thawed)–either use heparinized tubes or drop in directly
4. Invert tubes several times
5. Incubate in CO_2 incubator (5%) at 37°C for 72 hours. keeping caps loose
6. Every 24 hours. invert tubes
7. Add 0.2 ml of colecimid in each tube and place in incubator again for 2 hours.

8. Centrifuge tubes at 1000 rpm for 10 minutes
9. Remove supernatant with vacuum pump
10. Add 5 ml of hypotonic 0.075M KCl
11. Incubate tubes at 37°C, 5% CO_2 for 10 minutes
12. Centrifuge at 1000 rpm for 10 minutes at room temperature and remove supernatant
13. Add 5 ml of freshly prepared fixative, 7.5 mL of glacial acetic acid, 22.5 ml of methanol
14. Incubate tubes for 20 minutes at 37°C at 4.9% CO_2
15. Remove from incubator and resuspend pellet with Pasteur pipette
16. Centrifuge at 1000 rpm for 10 minutes and remove supernatant with vacuum pump
17. Add 5 ml of fixative to pellet
18. Incubate for 20 minutes (same as 15)
19. Remove from incubator, resuspend pellet, and centrifuge, remove supernatant, add fixative, and resuspend cells
20. Put in 4°C refrigeration.
21. Drop 3 drops of blood cell suspension from 24" on to a slide at 45° angle.
22. Mix staining solution:
    5 ml 10 mM K_2HPO_4
    1.5 ml Karyomax^R Giemsa stain
23. Flood slides with Giemsa staining solution and allow to sit for 20 minutes
24. Rinse by dipping slides in distilled water
25. De-stain slides for 10 minutes in 95% ethanol
26. Place slide in PBS (phosphate buffer saline) and incubate for 10 minutes at 56°C
27. Treat silde with 0.22 ml of 25% trypsin, 2.5 ml of methanol and 0.22 ml of stock Giemsa and 6.5 ml of PBS with a pH of 7.4.
28. Flood slide with stain solution for 15 minutes. Rinse with water and air dry
29. View slide under bright field, oil immersion microscope.

FISH

Fluorescence *in situ* hybridization (FISH) is a very sensitive technique that is used for detecting unusual chromosomal structural perturbation like deletions, transpositions, mutations, etc. Due to its sensitivity and precise localization information capabilities it is becoming a technique of wider choice. This technique relies on hybridization of a specific DNA probe which is labeled with a fluorescent tag which emits a characteristic color. By specific color development on the chromosome by virtue of DNA probe hybridization, the chromosome can be visualized with a confocal or a fluorescent microscope. The DNA probe can be designed such that it hybridizes only in normal chromosome and fails to hybridize in case a mutation is present on the chromosome (or vice versa). Hence by using just microscope chromosomal features predictive of various genetic disorders can be studied. A great number of companies now offer specialized FISH–kits for detecting abnormalities associated with specific diseases.

Herein under is described a whole chromosome painting protocol using whole chromosome coupled with a fluorescent dye. A whole chromosome probe is useful for detecting abnormal chromosomal structure.

Requirements

1. Ficoll–Paque
2. PBS buffer (137 mM NaCl; 8.1 mM $Na_2HPO_4.12H_2O$; 2.68 mM KCl; 1.47 mM KH_2PO_4, pH 7.4)
3. 10 × SSC buffer (1.5 M NaCl; 0.15 M sodium citrate)
4. 4% paraformaldehyde solution in PBS
5. Triton X–100
6. Nonidet P–40 (NP–40)
7. Saponin
8. Pepsin
9. Formamide
10. 0.1 M HCl
11. Chromosome painting probe labeled by Cy3
12. Anti–fade mounting medium.

Methodology

1. *Cell preparation*
   a. Isolate lymphocytes from heparinized human PBMCs using Ficoll–Paque according to manufacturer's instructions
   b. Smear the cells on a glass slide and immediately keep the slide in a coupling jar containing 4% paraformaldehyde for fixation for 5 minutes at RT.

c. Rinse slide with PBS for 5 minutes.
d. Permeablize the cells with freshly prepared Triton X–100/ Saponin (0.1%) solution. Perform twice at room temperature for 5 minutes each.
e. Rinse the slid with PBS. (If you are not developing the slide immediately, then it can be stored at this step for 1 week at 4°C).
f. Incubate the slide with pepsin (1 μg/ml) in 0.1 M HCl for 9 minutes at 37°C.
g. Wash with cold PBS for 1 minute.
h. Fix the slide again with 1% paraformaldehyde for 2–3 minutes at RT.
i. Wash with 2 × SSC for 5 minutes.

2. *FISH*
   a. Denature slides in 70% formamide in 2 × SSC solution at 65°C for 5 minutes.
   b. Prepare probe by taking 15 μl probe from tube and denature at 65°C for 5 minutes.
   c. Apply the denatured probe on the slide and cover the same with cover glass.
   d. Seal the slide with paper bond.
   e. Incubate at 42°C for 16 hours.
   f. Wash with 2 × SSC twice at 45°C for 5 minutes each
   g. Wash with 50% formamide/2 × SSC twice at 45°C for 5 minutes each.
   h. Wash with 0.1 × SSC at 45°C for 5 minutes
   i. Rinse slide with 4 × SSC containing 0.1% NP-40 at RT.
   j. Wash slide with PBS at room temperature for 5 minutes
   k. Counter stain the slide with Yo-Pro-1 at room temperature for 2–3 minutes.
   l. Wash the slide with PBS and mount in antifade mounting medium
   m. Examine the slide under fluorescent microscope.

RNA TECHNIQUES

RNA Isolation

Large amounts of very high quality total RNA in good yield can be obtained from adult organs. Any organ per se which is constantly secreting various proteins such as enzymes, structural proteins, etc. like pancreas, liver, etc. will yield a high amount of RNA. Unlike protein or DNA isolation, RNA isolation needs special precautions as RNase is present everywhere specially on the skin which can lead to degradation of RNA. Due to this reason, RNase should be removed from every reagent, plastic ware or glassware to be used in the purification. Diethyl pyrocarbonate (DEPC) is used for eradication of RNase from all ingredients used in RNA isolation. Gloves should be worn at all times to prevent any further contamination.

Reagents

1. TRIzol reagent
2. DEPC (diethyl pyrocarbonate)
3. DEPC treated H_2O: 0.05% DEPC, incubate at room temperature for at least 4 hours, then autoclave for 45 minutes at 121°C.
4. Chloroform
5. Isopropanol
6. Ethanol.

Methodology

1. Homogenize 100 mg tissue in 1 ml TRIzol reagent and let samples stand for 3 minutes at room temperature.
2. Add 0.2 ml chloroform/ml TRIzol, mix gently, let stand for 10 minutes at room temperature.
3. Centifuge at 14,000 rpm for 15 minutes at 4°C.
4. Transfer upper, clear part into new tubes.
5. 0.5 ml isopropanol/ml TRIzol, mix, room temperature for 10 minutes.
6. Centrifuge at 14,000 rpm for 10 minutes at 4°C.

7. Keep pellets, subject to 1ml 75% ethanol wash.
8. Air dry pellet for 10 minutes.
9. Dissolve pellets in proper amount DEPC treated H_2O.
10. Dilute 1.2 µl RNA into final 100 µl H_2O.
11. O.D. of the samples measured.
12. $O.D._{260}$ × 40 × (dilution factor) is µg/ ml RNA.

Note: 1. Typical yield from 100 mg brain tissue is roughly 80-100 µg.

2. OD_{260} of 40 µg RNA is 1.

PROTEIN TECHNIQUES

Protein Isolation

Unlike DNA or RNA isolation protein isolation is more basic technique and can be modified essentially on the basis of the type of downstream application desired from the isolated proteins. The isolation technique may differ slightly on this basis besides differing on the basis of organism from which the protein needs to be isolated. It is considerably easy to isolate proteins (or DNA or RNA) from eukaryotic/mammalian cells rather than from bacterial cells/microorganisms because of the presence of a rigid cell wall on them which is absent in eukaryotes.

Like DNA or RNA isolation, protein isolation procedures also need to address the problems associated with proteases which can lead to degradation of valuable protein samples. A number of protease inhibitors are commercially available and are used in all the reagents used during protein isolation. Such compounds include PMSF (phenyl methyl sulphonyl fluoride), EDTA, DTT (Dithiothreitol, a potent reducing agent), aprotinin, leupeptatin and pepstatin. Besides these isolated inhibitory compounds, many companies like Roche, Sigma, etc. sell readymade protease inhibitor cocktails which can take care of nearly all known proteases.

Broadly, all the isolation protocols emphasize on use of protease inhibitors and processing of samples at 4°C to avoid any kind of degradation and loss of activity of the protein constituents. This is very important when activity of any enzyme from the lysate needs to be analyzed. Table 12.1 provides a broad description various cell lysis protocols in use. Two basic protocols for protein extractions, first one is directed towards isolation of protein from prokaryotes and the second one from mammalian cells are described.

Experiment I

Isolation of soluble proteins from cultured Escherichia coli.

Requirements

1. Pure *E. coli* strain

Table 12.1: Various methodologies used to lyse cells for protein extraction

Technique	*Application*	*General procedure*
Osmotic lysis-This very gentle method is well suited for applications in which the lysate needs subcellular fractionation.	Blood cells, tissue culture cells	Suspend cells in a hypo-osmotic solution.
Freeze-thaw lysis-Many types of cells can be lysed by subjecting them to one or more cycles of quick freezing and subsequent thawing.	Bacterial cells, tissue culture cells	Rapidly freeze cell suspension using liquid nitrogen, then thaw. Repeat if necessary.
Detergent lysis-Detergents solubilize cellular membranes, lysing cells and liberating their contents	Tissue culture cells	Suspend cells in lysis solution containing detergent.
Enzymatic lysis-Cells with cell walls can be lysed gently fol- (lyso- lowing enzymatic removal of the cell wall. This must be done with an enzyme specific for the type of cell to be lysed	Plant tissue, bacterial cells, fungal cells	Treat cells with enzyme in iso-osmotic solution zyme for bacterial cells, cellulase and pectinase for plant cells, lyticase for yeast cells).
Sonication-Ultrasonic waves generated by a sonicator lyse cells through shear forces. Complete shearing is obtained when maximal agitation is achieved, (minimize heating and foaming).	Cell suspensions	Sonicate cell suspension in short bursts to avoid heating. Cool on ice between bursts.
French pressure cell-Cells are lysed by shear forces resulting from forcing cell suspension through a small orifice under high pressure.	Microorganisms with cell walls (bacteria, algae, yeasts)	Place cell suspension in chilled French pressure cell. Apply pressure and collect extruded lysate.
Grinding-Some cell types can be opened by hand grinding with a mortar and pestle.	Solid tissues, microorganisms	Tissue or cells are normally frozen with liquid nitrogen and ground to a fine powder. Alumina or sand may aid grinding.
Homogenization with beads (bead beating)-The abrasive actions of the vortexed beads break cell walls, liberating cellular costituents including proteins.	Cell suspensions,	Suspend cells in an equal volume of chilled lysis solution and place into a sturdy tube. Add 1–3 grams of chilled glass beads per gram of wet cells. Vortex 1 minute and incubate cells on ice 1 minute. Repeat vortexing and chilling two to four times.

2. Growth media–Luria Bertani medium (autoclaved and preferably in a flask)
3. PBS
4. Sonicator or a bead beater.

Methodology

1. Aseptically inoculate the *E. coli* in growth media and allow it to grow at 37°C for 16–20 hours.
2. Pellet the culture by centrifugation at 5000 rpm for 20 minutes at 4°C.
3. Discard the supernatant and wash the pellet by resuspending the pellet in 1/10th culture volume of PBS (perform this and all the subsequent steps on ice only).
4. Repeat centrifugation (step 2) and discard PBS.
5. Resuspend the pellete in 1/100th volume of PBS.
6. Lyse the cells by mechanical lysis using either a sonicator or a mini-bead beator.
   a. Sonication–transfer the lysate to a 15 ml conical tube (use only polypropylene tube) and subject to sonication using a 'microtip' (sonication probe meant for giving high frequency sound pulses in low volumes. The ultrasonic pulses lead to generation of sonic voids which leads to rupturing of cell wall and membrane). Pulse the sample with 30 seconds pulses at 20 W followed by 30 seconds incubation on ice. Repeat the sonication cycle 3 times. At all times keep the sample on ice and avoid frothing.
   [**Caution**–Do not come in direct contact with probe while sonicating or immediately after sonication].
   b. Bead beating–Transfer the lysate (approx. 1 ml) to a 2 ml screw cap tube supplied with the bead beater and fill up the tube with equal volume of 0.5 mm Zircon–silica beads pre wetted with PBS (in place of 0.5 mm, 0.1 mm or 1 mm beads can also be used). Subject sample to beating in the beater at maximum speed for 1 minute, followed by incubation on ice for 1 minute. Repeat this beating cycle three times (if 1 mm beads are used then give 4-5 pulses and 2-3 pulses only for 0.1 mm beads). Centrifuge the tube at low speed, 2000 rpm for 2-3 minutes at 4°C and collect the lysate.

7. Centrifuge the lysate at 12000 rpm for 20 minutes at 4°C. Collect the clarified lysate at chilled tubes and store in aliquots at -20°C or -70°C.

Experiment II

Isolation of proteins from cultured cells.

Requirements

1. Cultured cells
2. Deionized water
3. PBS

Methodology

1. Transfer the cells by resuspending them in PBS to a microcentrifuge tube
2. Pellet the culture by centrifugation at 5000 rpm for 20 minutes at 4°C.
3. Discard the supernatant and resuspend the pellet in water and incubate on ice for 15–20 minutes for osmotic lysis.
4. Centrifugation at 12000 rpm at 4°C for 20 minutes to remove cell debris and store ther supernatant containing the proteins and store in aliquots at -20° or -70°C.

Alternate protocol (detergent based lysis):

Requirements:

1. Lysis buffer: 10 ml 10% sodium dodecyl sulphate (SDS)
   10 ml glycerol
   10 ml β-mercaptoethanol
   8 ml 0.5 M Tris pH 6.8
   1 ml 0.1% bromophenol blue
   51 ml H_2O
2. PBS

Methodology

1. Spin down 10^6 cells and wash, if required, in phosphate buffered saline.
2. Resuspend cells in 100 µl warmed lysis buffer, vortex then boil for 5-10 minutes to break up DNA.

3. Cool (not on ice-the SDS will precipitate) and centrifuge to collect droplets.
4. Vortex briefly to mix.
5. The samples may now be analyzed by SDS-PAGE and western blotting, or store samples at -20°C until required.

Protein Estimation

Immediate process which needs to be performed after protein isolation is to estimate the yield of protein obtained so that a known amount of protein can be used in all the subsequent applications like ELISA, western blotting or in specialized studies like interaction analysis.

Proteins are the most abundant biomolecules, constituting more than 50% of the dry weight of the cell and they are known to perform many different biological functions. Thus, besides protein isolation, estimation of total protein in various body fluids is also critical from point of view of a biochemist. Qualitative and quantitative estimation of proteins in biological fluids is based on the physicochemical properties of proteins.

Proteins react with a variety of reagents to form colored products, which can be measured calorimetrically. They are important for qualitative and quantitative estimation of protein and their constituent amino acids. Depending upon the sensitivity of various assays various protocols have been developed and employed over the years. A few of those methods used for protein estimation are described below:

1. *Ninhydrin method.* It is one of the most important reactions used for the qualitative detection of hydrolytic products of protein i.e. amino acids. All α-amino acids (excluding proline) react with ninhydrin (triketohydrindene hydrate) at ambient temperature between pH 4 and 8 to give a blue/purple-colored compound, which intensifies to deep purple on heating. A spectrophotometric reading at 570 nm gives an estimation of amount of amino acids present in the sample. Proline and hydroxyproline forms a yellow colored complex, hence they are read at 440 nm.

   Reaction principle:

Ninhydrin + Amino acid → L -hydrindantin + Aldehyde + CO_2 + NH_3

Ninhydrin + Hydrindantin + NH_3 → Purple colored complex
(Ruhemann's purple)

2. *Biuret method.* When urea is heated to 180°C it forms biuret which in the presence of strong alkali reacts with dilute solutions of copper

sulfate to form a violet colored complex. Proteins and peptides give this reaction. Presence of at least two peptide bonds is essential for the reaction. Proteins give violet or purple color while proteoses and peptones give light pink color. Histidine gives a positive biuret reaction. Two or more–$CONH_2$ groups joined directly or though a carbon or nitrogen atom give this reaction.

Absorption maximum of the colored complex is 540 nm. Since the method is based on reaction with peptide bonds, it is an absolute one. The main disadvantage is its lack of sensitivity. It cannot be used to estimate protein less than 1 mg/ ml. Amino acids and dipeptides do not give this reaction. The intensity of the color produced is proportional to the amount of protein undergoing the reaction.

3. *Bradford's method.* The principle is similar to the biuret test as described above, however, it is much more sensitive. The principle is that when the dye Coomassie Brilliant Blue G-250 (in acidic solution) binds to proteins it turns a deep blue color (technically, its absorption maximum shifts from 465 to 595 nm) and the amount of dye bound is proportional to the amont of protein present. The Bradford's assay is thus a quantitative test for protein. This method is simple and very sensitive. Colour development is rapid but not very stable.
4. *Lowry's method.* This is also a very sensitive method. It involves the formation of a copper-protein complex in alkaline solution and the reduction of phosphotungstic and phosphomolybdic acids by the copper-protein complex into tungsten blue and molybdenum blue respectively. Absorption maxima-660 nm. Sensitivity is 1 pg/ml.
5. *BCA method.* The method utilizes bicinchoninic acid (BCA) as the detection reagent for Cu^{1+}, which is formed when Cu^{2+} is reduced by protein in an alkaline environment. A purple-colored reaction product is formed by the chelation of two molecules of BCA with one cuprous ion (Cu^{1+}). This water-soluble complex exhibits a strong absorbance at 562 nm that is linear with increasing protein concentrations. The macromolecular structure of protein, the number of peptide bonds and the presence of four amino acids (cysteine, cystine, tryptophan and tyrosine) are reported to be responsible for color formation with BCA. Studies with di-, tri- and tetrapeptides suggest that the extent of color formation is caused by more than the mere sum of individual color-producing functional groups.

Table 12.2: Comparison of various protein estimation methods

Method	*Detection range*	*Compatibility/Application*	*Protocol*	*Interfering agent*
UV absorbance	0.1–1 OD_{280}/ ml	Only for purified proteins with known absorbance factor	Read absorbance 280 nm.	Nucleic acid, detergents, cofactors, phenolic compounds, pigments, reducing agents, etc
Lowry's method	10 μg/ml-1 mg/ml	Very accurate	1 ml reagent + 0.2 ml sample. Incubate 10' RT. Add 0.1 ml Folin-Ciocalteu. Incubate 30' RT. Read 750 nm	Many detergents, reducing agents, EDTA, GuHCl, $(NH_4)_2SO_4$, >0.1M Tris.
Bradford's method	1-1500 μg/ml	For quick estimation where accuracy is not important	Reagent + various volumes sample. Vortex and read 595 nm	Detergents
BCA method	0.5-20 μg/ml	Compatible with proteins solubilized with detergents, Chaotropic agents. Proteins on affinity supports. Sugars, DNA, protease inhibitors.	2 ml reagent + 0.1 ml sample. Incubation 30 min., 37ºC. Read 562 nm	Reducing agents
Biuret method	1-10 mg/ml	Very accurate and simple	Read 550 nm	Glucose, Ammonium sulfate, Sulfhydryl compounds, PO_4 buffers

Protein Fractionation

Once the proteins have been isolated and estimated, they need to be separated and different proteins differ in terms of their molecular size, charge and shape. Hence, using these variable features, they can be separated using various techniques on the following basis which can depend on any of their specific features:

1. Molecular size
2. Solubility
3. Electrical charge
4. Adsorption properties
5. Specific bioaffinity–specialized feature of certain proteins.

On the basis of these criteria many techniques for protein purification have been developed and are in use, but the emphasis here is on some of the most popular procedures and the principles involved in their use.

Differential Centrifugation

Using the typical crude cell 'lysate' containing disrupted cell membranes, cellular organelles and a large number of soluble proteins, all dispersed in an aqueous buffered solution, the membranes and the organelles can be separated from the soluble proteins by differential centrifugation.

This type of centrifugation involves the use of different centrifugal 'g' force (rpm) for different durations of time. For example if the protein of interest is in the mitochondrial fraction, the crude cell lysate is first centrifuged at 4000 g for removing nuclei, debris, etc. The supernatant contains among other elements the mitochondria which can be pelleted at 15,000 g for 20 minutes.

Salt Fractionation

Proteins show a variation in solubility, that depends on the concentration of salts in the solution. This method is frequently used to separate serum proteins into albumins and globulins. Albumin is soluble in water whereas globulins are not. Globulins are soluble in weak salt solutions, going into solution at salt concentrations of 0.1 mol/L. This phenomenon called "Salting In" because presence of salt enhances the solubility. This is due to the electrostatic attraction between the salt ions and the charged groups of the protein molecules, which decreases the attraction of protein molecules for each other.

Alternatively, as the salt concentration increases, the salt ions compete for the water molecules of the hydrated polar groups of the proteins so that the proteins become dehydrated and less soluble-the phenomenon of "Salting Out", wherein the protein is brought out of solution by adding salt. Each protein has a characteristic salting out point based on the its characteristic water molecule requirement to maintain soluble status. Ammonium sulfate is most commonly used for salt fractionation.

Western Transfer

One of the major advances in protein analysis has been the development of techniques of resolved proteins from polyacrylamide gels (discussed in section I.5.) onto a thin support matrix for further analysis. One of the most common matrices used for this purpose is nitrocellulose membrane, to which they are immobilized irreversibly. The technique of electrophoretic transfer of proteins from SDS–polyacrylamide gel to this solid matrix is termed as western blotting. This technique of protein analysis is highly advantageous over PAGE because of many reasons such as (i) the protein binds to the matrix in an unhindered manner, i.e. matrix does not hamper the protein accessibility, hence many downstream applications can be performed which are otherwise not possible, (ii) time required for downstream processing is much less, (iii) ease of handling compared to gels and (iv) the proteins once transferred on the membrane can be stored for longer duration without any loss of activity.

A variety of matrices can be used for these applications, which includes nitrocellulose membrane, charged and uncharged nylon membrane, specialized coated matrices such as PVDF nitro cellulose membrane (which has the advantage over the conventional membrane it terms of sensitivity and processing time required). Once the proteins are transferred on the membrane, they can be visualized by reversible staining prior to analysis of the transferred proteins by either immunoblotting or N–terminal protein sequencing.

Requirements

1. Proteins resolved on SDS-PAGE

2. Transfer buffer (Tris base, 48 mM; Glycine, 39 mM; SDS, 0.03%; Methanol, 20%)
3. Nitrocellulose membrane (never touch the membrane with bare hands)
4. Ponceau solution (Ponceau–S, 2 g and acetic acid, 10% for 100 ml
5. Deionized water.

Methodology (Semi–dry transfer Method)

1. Resolve the proteins on the SDS–PAGE gel as mentioned earlier in chapter 8 (the percentage of gel should be considered carefully here, as large proteins do not transfer properly from gels of higher percentage. The recommended percentage for proteins upto 15 kDa is 15%; 15 to 60 kDa–12.5 and 10% for proteins above 60 kDa).
2. Soak the resolved gel in transfer buffer for 20–30 minutes.
3. Soak nitrocellulose membrane and Whatman filter sheets of the size of gel in transfer buffer.
4. Prepare the transfer sandwich as below on the transfer apparatus:
   Negative electrode
   Three layers of Whatman paper
   Presoaked gel
   Nitrocellulose membrane
   3 layers of Whatman paper
   Positive electrode
5. Roll out the air bubbles from the sandwich using a pipette (presence of air bubbles interfere with transfer as it generates a no conductance area; hence no protein is transferred in those regions).
6. Transfer proteins from gel onto the membrane using current at 0.8 mA/cm^2 for 1 hour.
7. Remove the transfer sandwich after the transfer and separate the membrane with transferred proteins from the gel.
8. Briefly soak the membrane in Ponceau solution (1 minute) and remove the excess solution.
9. Wash repeatedly with deionized water till red/pink bands on a colorless white background are visible.
10. Record the profile and air dry the membrane and store in folds of filter paper at 4°C till further use.

Part—III:

Analysis of Various Specimens

After various techniques or tricks of the biochemistry laboratory have been understood and tried out, the very next step is to apply them in actual 'field' conditions and see the results.

There is nothing more intriguing than to see the theory turn to practicality

As a clinical biochemist various types and natures of clinical samples come for investigations. Sometimes the investigations asked by the physicians are the most obvious and sometimes most extraordinary, but such too routine or out–of–routine testing should not be taken lightly and quality control aspect mentioned earlier should be practiced all the time. Please note that though some technique might become 'too' routine, do not undermine the safety aspect at any instance and follow proper guidelines for disposing body fluids/ extracts.

13

Analysis of Blood

"Blood–The Fluid of Life"

The statement holds more facts than mere fiction of medicine. As the carrier of components needed in every process of human body, the health status of blood is very good indication of physiology of whole body. Most blood tests fall within one of two categories: *screening* or *diagnostic*.

Screening tests are used to detect a disease when there is little or no evidence that a person has a suspected disease. For example, measuring cholesterol levels helps to identify one of the risks of heart disease. These screening tests are performed on people who may show no symptoms of heart disease, as a tool for the physician to detect a potentially harmful and evolving condition. In order for screening tests to be the most useful they must be readily available, accurate, inexpensive, pose little risk, and cause little discomfort to the patient. Against this diagnostic tests are utilized when a specific disease is suspected by the physician and the test is essentially performed to verify the presence and the severity of that disease.

GLUCOSE ESTIMATION AND GLUCOSE TOLERANCE TEST

Quantitative estimation of glucose in blood has become virtually the most routine in clinical practice; especially it is used for screening and following up of metabolic disorders like *Diabetes mellitus*. Homeostasis of glucose, which involves maintenance of blood glucose levels involves a complex process, which is initiated from glucose uptake by the tissues, then glycolysis, glyconeogenesis, glycogenolysis, etc. It is regulated by the critical interplay of various hormones on metabolic enzymes. This is necessary because vital tissues like brain survive principally by taking glucose from the blood. Any derangement in the process leads to either high level of glucose in the blood called hyperglycemia or low level called hypoglycemia, both the conditions being detrimental for health, the latter being a more serious condition which might lead to failure of brain function and might lead to coma.

A panoply of hormones have been implicated in regulating the glucose homeostasis like insulin, which is the only hormone which brings down the high blood sugar levels and other counter regulatory hormones like glucagon, corticosteroids, thyroid hormones, growth hormones, noradrenaline, adrenaline, etc. increase the levels.

Presence of high levels of glucose in urine results when blood glucose level is high (180 mg/ml) and renal threshold is exceeded. Such a condition is called as glycosuria which leads to polyuria in patients of *Diabetes mellitus*. This disease results from under production of insulin or excessive production of counter hormones like glucagons, thyroid hormones, adrenaline, corticosteroids, etc.

Quantitative estimation of sugar is done with whole blood, plasma or serum and several methods have been in use. But before coming to the techniques of blood sugar estimation and its implications, it is important to get acquainted with various terminologies critical in glucose monitoring tests.

Terminologies

Blood sugar. Generally means blood glucose. Certain reducing substances like glutathione (present in red cell membrane), glucuronic acid, threonine, uric acid, ascorbic acid, fructose, etc. give erroneously high values when any alkaline copper reduction method is adopted. So care is taken to avoid interference by these substances by certain modification of the techniques.

True glucose. When glucose estimation is done by enzymatic methods, e.g. glucose oxidase or hexokinase methods to obtain actual glucose values.

Fasting blood sugar. Fasting is defined as no caloric intake for at least 8 hours preceding the measurement. A fasting plasma glucose level of 126 mg/dl or greater is one of the diagnostic criteria for *Diabetes mellitus*.

Postprandial blood sugar (PPBS). Blood sample is collected 2 hours after the ingestion of a meal. Plasma glucose of 200 mg/dl or greater after 2 hours of ingestion of oral glucose diagnoses *Diabetes mellitus*.

Random sampling. Blood is collected any time without prior preparation of the patient (either fast or a meal, etc.). Symptoms of diabetes with random blood glucose more than or equal to 200 mg/dl also defines *Diabetes mellitus*.

Collection of Blood Sample

Blood is usually collected from a vein into a bottle containing a mixture of potassium ethylene diamine tetra acetate (EDTA) and sodium fluoride at a ratio 1 : 2 (w/w). Five mg of the mixture is adequate for 2 ml of blood. The tube should be gently but thoroughly shaken for complete mixing. Both the substances act as anticoagulant and NaF prevents glycolysis in RBCs and WBCs by inhibiting the enzyme enolase. Fluoride can interfere with some glucose oxidase techniques. To avoid glycolysis the sample can be centrifuged and the plasma separated from the cells.

Detection of Blood Glucose-Principle

A. *Enzymatic methods:*

i. *Glucose oxidase method:* Glucose oxidase catalyses the oxidation of glucose (which is present in the plasma) to gluconic acid and hydrogen peroxide. The hydrogen peroxide is estimated (indirectly) colorimetrically in the presence of peroxidase that catalyses transfer of oxygen from peroxide (H_2O_2) to chromogenic oxygen acceptor such as orthotoluidine or orthodianisidine or 4–aminophenazone converting them to colored compounds. It is the most widely used protocol for glucose estimation as of today. In case of the compound 4–aminophenazone, oxygen is taken up by it and together with phenol, it forms a pink colored chromogen which can be measured at 515 nm.

$$\text{Glucose} \xrightarrow[\text{Oxidase}]{\text{Glucose}} \text{Gluconolactone} + O_2 \xrightarrow{H_2O} \text{Gluconic acid} + H_2O_2$$

$$\underset{\text{(chromogenic receivers)}}{H_2O_2 + 4\text{–aminophenazone}} \xrightarrow{\text{Peroxidase}} \underset{\text{(Pink)}}{\text{colored compound} + H_2O}$$

ii. *Hexokinase method:* Hexokinase acts in the following way:

$$\text{Glucose} + \text{ATP} \xrightarrow{\text{Hexokinase}} \text{Glucose-6-phosphate} + \text{ADP} + \text{Pi (G-6-P)}$$

$$\text{G-6-P} + \text{NAD}^+ \xrightarrow{\text{G-6-P-dehydrogenase}} 6\ \text{phosphogluconate} + \text{NADH} + \text{H}^+$$

The rate of formation of NADH is followed spectrophotometrically at 340 nm.

B. *Reduction methods:*

i. *Alkaline copper reduction methods:* Reducing sugars in hot alkaline medium produce enediols which are strong reducing agents that can convert Cu^{2+} ions to Cu^+ ions which combine with OH^- ions to form yellow CuOH which upon heating is converted to red Cu_2O. Cu_2O produced in the reaction is proportional to the amount of reducing sugar that is present in the solution. When phosphomolybdic acid (or arsenomolybdic acid reagent) is added at the last step, the oxidation of Cu^+ to Cu^{2+} is coupled to reduction of the acid to molybdenum blue, which can be estimated colorimetrically.

Glucose Estimation by Glucose Oxidase Method

Requirements

1. Phosphate buffer (PBS): 100 mmol/l, pH 7.0
2. Color reagent: To 100 ml of the above phosphate buffer add the following in the order and then mix to dissolve. 4-aminophenazone,

16 mg; glucose oxidase (GOD), 1800 units; peroxidase (POD), 100 units; Phenol, 105 mg and Tween-20, 50 ml. Both GOD and POD enzymes can be reconstituted in PBS and stored at 4°C in brown bottles.

3. Benzoic acid–1g/L
4. Glucose standard solution–100 mg/dL.

Methodology

1. Prepare standard glucose tubes in glass test tubes in total 2 ml of water. Glucose volumes from 0.1 to 0.5 ml (1–5 mg glucose as quality control pool-QC). Take 0.1 ml of test sample in duplicate for estimation. The final volume should be 2 ml. In parallel take two tubes wherein no glucose or test sample has been added for quality control.
2. Add 1.2 ml of color reagent in all tubes and incubate at 37°C water bath for 15 minutes after mixing the contents thoroughly. In one tube mix 1.2 ml of color reagent with 0.1 ml water (this would serve as blank reaction tube in the colorimetric estimation for background correction).
3. Remove tubes from waterbath and cool to room temperature. Set the spectrophotometer to zero using blank at 510 nm and measure the absorbance of glucose standards, test samples and control tubes.
4. Calculation and calibration graph
   Plot the standard graph with glucose amount plotted as a function (against) of absorbance. Calculate the amount of glucose in the test sample using this graph and calculate the glucose amount/dl of blood. The measurable range in this graph is 10–500 mg/dl.

Reliability and Interference of the Test

Since glucose is the most common analyte measured in a laboratory, it is advisable to include an internal QC (normal QC pool) with every batch of samples analysed in the day, irrespective of the number of samples in a batch. Further, even when a single sample is analysed as an "emergency" sample at any time of the day or night, it is essential to include an internal QC. From the QC results obtained for the day, mean, standard deviation and % CV can be calculated to ensure that within-day precision is well within the acceptable limit, i.e. 5%.

Any sample that gives a glucose value more than 500 mg/dl should be diluted 1:2 with 0.9 g% sodium chloride solution and the correct value obtained by multiplying the result by 3. At high plasma levels, uric acid, glutathione and bilirubin may interfere with the assay by causing a decrease in glucose values. Ascorbic acid will decrease glucose values by retarding color development

Alternate methodology-Astoor and King's method

Methodology

1. Place 0.1 ml of blood in a centrifuge tube.
2. Add 3.8 ml of isotonic sodium sulphate—copper sulphate solution and mix.
3. Add 0.1 ml of sodium tungstate solution and mix.
4. Centrifuge at 2000 rpm for 10. Take three tubes labeled 'T (test)', 'S (standard)' and 'B (blank)' and take 1 ml of supernatant standard glucose (0.125 mmol/L) and isotonic solution respectively.
5. Add 1 ml of alkaline tartrate solution to all the tubes, place them in a boiling water bath for 10 m and then add 3 ml each of arsenomolybdic acid reagent and distilled water to the tubes.
6. Read at 670 nm.

Calculations

$$\frac{T-B}{S-B} \times \frac{4}{0.1} \times 0.125 \text{ mmol/l}$$

Diagnostic values

Condition	*Sampling at*	*Glucose concentration (mg/dl)*	
		Venous	*Capillary*
Diabetes mellitus			
	Fasting	≥ 120	> 120
	PP	> 180	> 200
Impaired glucose tolerance			
	Fasting	< 120	< 120
	PP (2 hours after food)	< 120–180	< 140–200

Clinical Relevance

In a country like India where 1–2% population is known to suffer from diabetes, it becomes a severe medical problem, which needs immediate attention. Diabetes or hyperglycemia is clinically the condition when plasma glucose level is equal to or exceeds 110 mg/dl during fasting conditions or 2 hours postprandial glucose level equal to or exceeds 140 mg/dl on more than one occasion. Though the cases of hypoglycemia are relatively rare, it is still a critical medical condition because its effects are more life-threatening than hyperglycemia. Clinically when blood glucose levels fall below 50 mg/dl it is considered as hypoglycemia.

Causes of Hyperglycemia

1. Deficiency or under response to insulin–*Diabetes mellitus*, obesity, etc.
2. Hyperactivity of hormones that raise blood glucose like thyroxine, cortisol, adrenaline, growth hormone, glucagon, etc.
3. Diseases of pancreas like pancreatitis, etc.
4. Drugs like thiazide diuretics, glucocorticoids.
5. Miscellaneous conditions like congenital rubella, genetic diseases like Down's syndrome, anesthesia, stress, etc.
6. Gestational *Diabetes mellitus*.

Causes of Hypoglycemia

1. Overdose of insulin during treatment of diabetes.
2. Drug induced (other than insulin), e.g. oral hypoglycemic agents.
3. Hypofunction of thyroid, pituitary and adrenal cortex.
4. Starvation, severe exercise.

Glucose Tolerance Test (GTT)

Glucose tolerance test is defined as the capacity of the body to tolerate an extraload of glucose. This test is useful in *Diabetes mellitus* in borderline cases and diabetes in pregnancy.

After overnight fasting a fasting blood sugar is measured and 75 g of glucose is given to the patient for ingestion. 2 hours after the ingestion of oral glucose again a blood sample is taken and glucose estimated. When the plasma glucose level is 200 mg/dl or more, then a diagnosis of diabetes is established.

Precautions to be taken when doing a GTT. The patient should not be stressed, should not smoke, physical activity should not be restricted and the daily carbohydrate intake should be greater than 150 g. For diabetes in pregnancy a different GTT procedure and criteria is used to diagnose.

Interpretation of GTT

In a normal individual, blood glucose levels start immediately after glucose ingestion with peak reaching within 1 hour (160–170 mg/dl) and then the levels start to fall off. At the end of 2 hours the blood glucose levels reaches the normal status. At all these stages the urine glucose is absent in the individual.

Extended GTT. Instead of ending at 2 hours after taking glucose, the blood glucose is measured half hourly for upto 4-5 hours. This is to know how the curve behaves below the normal fasting glucose limits. This test is performed in some conditions causing hypoglycemia.

In a person having a predisposition to diabetes or has a suspected case, the time gap between glucose ingestion and normalization of blood glucose levels is more than two hours. The wider the time for normalization, less the tolerance to glucose and consequently higher chances of developing diabetes later. Though such a testing is not in use any longer for diagnosis of diabetes and an extended GTT is though used sometimes to detect reactive hypoglycemia. But even in such cases the blood glucose levels need to be correlated with physiological symptoms, because according to the test parameters almost 25% of the individuals would turn out to be hypoglycemics but since they report no symptoms associated with hypoglycemia they are considered as negatives. Some typical extended GTT curves may look as follows:

Early diabetes : normal fasting glucose, glucose high during the first 2 hour indicating diabetes, low plasma glucose hours 3 to 4.

Postgastrectomy : rapid elevation of glucose by 1 hour, rapid decline with a trough at 2 to 3 hours.

Idiopathic hypoglycemia : normal plasma glucose hours 1 and 2, low glucose hour 3, return to baseline by hour 5.

Idiopathic postprandial syndrome : Have postprandial adrenergic symptoms with normal GTT.

Impaired fasting glucose. When fasting blood glucose levels are between 110–125 mg/dl, it is defined as impaired fasting glucose.

Impaired glucose tolerance. When blood glucose levels are between 140–199 mg/dl after 2 hours of ingestion of 75 mg of oral glucose.

Cortisone stressed GTT. This test is carried out to detect latent diabetes in which patient is stressed by administering cortisone before carrying out the GTT.

Intravenous GTT. It is primarily done when vomiting occurs after administration of glucose orally or oral GTT curve is flat. In such cases, 20% solution of glucose are infused until 0.5 gm of glucose/kg of body weight. Blood samples are taken at 30, 60, 90 and 120 minutes. Normally peak occurs within 30 minutes after infusion and returns to normal after 90.

URIC ACID

Uric acid is a 2, 6, 8-trihydroxypurine and exists in keto and enol forms and is the major end product of metabolism of purine nucleosides, adenosine and guanosine. In most mammals with exception of human beings, an enzyme uricase converts the insoluble uric acid to a more soluble compound allantoin. But in humans, 75% of uric acid is excreted in urine through kidney, wherein it is filtrated through glomerulus preferably in the form of soluble salt (urate). Rest of the 25% uric acid is excreted through bile, intestinal and gastric secretions. The uric acid which is secreted in gastric intestinal tract is broken down by intestinal bacteria by a process called as uricolysis. Since, uric acid is poorly soluble in water, its accumulation in can lead to renal damage and gout.

Source of uric acid. The purines–adenine and guanine are used in body for synthesis of nucleic acids (DNA or RNA). Purines can be either derived from various dietary sources through catabolism of nucleic acids or they can be synthesized *de novo.* The purines taken up in the diet can either used for synthesis of nucleic acids or they are oxidized into uric acid. Adenine oxidizes to hypoxanthine, which further oxidized to xanthine. Guanine is also oxidized to xanthine. This xanthine is converted to uric acid by enzyme xanthine oxidase.

Sample Collection

Early morning blood should be collected. Purine rich diet should be avoided in the night just before the day of collection. The blood sample should be used as early as possible because bacteria breakdown uric acid on long-term storage. Thymol, an antibacterial agent, can be added as preservative. Serum or plasma can be used for estimation as well.

Methods of Estimation

Principle

The methods are essentially based on its reducing activity at alkaline pH through its oxidation to allantoin or its specific degradation to allantoin and hydrogen peroxide through enzyme uricase.

Caraway's method. Phosphotungstic acid in alkaline medium oxidizes uric acid to allantoin and itself gets reduced to "tungsten blue" which is measured colorimetrically at 700 nm.

Requirements

1. Sodium tungstate solution–10% solution
2. Sulphuric acid–0.33 mol/l
3. Tungstinic acid solution–Add 50 ml sodium tungstate solution + 50 ml sulphuric acid in total 800 ml water with slow mixing.
4. Phosphotungstate solution–To 50 g of sodium tungstate dissolved in 400 ml water, slowly add 40 ml orthophosphoric acid. Cool and make volume to 500 ml. Dilute 1: 10 with water before use.
5. Sodium carbonate—10% solution in water
6. Urate standard.

Methodology

1. In a centrifuge tube add 0.6 ml of serum and 5.4 ml of tungstic acid.
2. Mix well and centrifuge at 2000 rpm for 10 minutes.
3. Use the supernatant for the assay and setup the reaction as follows

Additive	*Test*	*Standard*	*Blank*
Supernatant	3.0 ml	–	–
Distilled water	–	–	3.0 ml
Urate standard (0.84 mg/ml)	–	3.0 ml	–
Sodium carbonate	0.6 ml	0.6 ml	0.6 ml
Phosphotungstate	0.6 ml	0.6 ml	0.6 ml

4. Mix well and keep for 30 minutes at room temperature.
5. Measure absorbance at 670 nm.

Calculations

Serum urate = OD of test/OD of standard × 8.4 mg per 100 ml

Levels of uric acid. The urate pool in the body is about 1.2 g in men and 600 mg in women and there is turnover of about 0.4 g daily. Fresh meat, poultry and fish are rich sources of purines in the diet which contribute another 300 mg.

By contrast, patients with gouty arthritis and tissue deposition of urate may have a urate pool as large as 18,000 to 30,000 mg. Over production of uric acid may result from increased synthesis of purine precursors.

Normal serum levels of uric acid:

2.5-6.2 mg in females
4.5-8.0 mg/dl in male.

Clinical Relevance

Disturbances in levels of uric acid:

A. *Hyperuricemia (>7 mg/dl in male and >6 mg/dl in female)*
1. Decreased excretion in urine: Renal disorder
2. Increased production of uric acid–Primary cause includes HGPRT deficiency (enzymes which converts the residual pool of xanthine, the uric acid precursor into nucleic acid analogs), PRPP synthetase over activity, G-6-phosphatase deficiency, adenosine deaminase deficiency. Secondary causes include polycythemia vera, chronic lymphocytic leukemia, psoriasis, etc.

B. *Hypouricemia (less than 2 mg/dl)*
1. Enzyme deficiency, e.g.: Xanthine oxidase
2. Decreased reabsorption in the kidney because of renal tubular diseases like Fanconis syndrome
3. Decreased synthesis because of liver diseases
4. Drugs: 6-mercaptopurine, azathioprine inhibits *de novo* purine synthesis leading to hypouricemia.

C. *Gout* It is one of the common clinical manifestations of hyperuricemia. When monosodium urate precipitates from supersaturated body fluids and the deposits of urate are responsible for the observed clinical signs and symptoms. It is not a single disorder but a group of disorders, which in their full development are manifested by:
1. An increase in the serum urate concentration
2. Recurrent attacks of a characteristic type of acute arthritis in which crystals of monosodium urate monohydrate are demonstrable in the leukocytes of synovial fluid.
3. Aggregated deposits of monosodium urate monohydrate crystals chiefly in and around the joints of the extremities are cartilages, bursa, subcutaneous tissues (tophi).

4. Renal disease involving interstitial tissues and blood vessels.
5. Uric acid nephrolithiasis.

In an acute attack of gout, the plasma urate level rises to a maximum of about 15 mg/dl. In chronic gout, the plasma urate level usually remains in high normal range. In many cases of gout, the causes of the raised serum levels cannot be ascertained. Estimation of plasma urate is important principally for diagnosis and monitoring of gout and toxemia of pregnancy.

PROTEINS ANALYSIS

Serum proteins are generally classified as *albumins* and *globulins*. Globulins are the proteins precipitated by half saturation of a solution with ammonium sulphate, while albumins are precipitated on fully saturating the solution.

Albumin is synthesized and secreted by the liver cells into plasma. It is the most abundant and most homogenous of serum proteins. Each molecule is a single polypeptide of 69 kilo Daltons and has a large number of cationic and anionic groups, with a net negative charge at physiological pH (7.4). Thus it can complex with a variety of anionic substances in blood and acts as a general carrier protein; e.g. fatty acid anions and acetylated amino acids. Albumin plays a significant role in maintaining plasma osmotic pressure, because it stays in the intravascular compartment, unlike smaller, diffusible molecules, and does not diffuse out into the interstitial fluid.

The globulin fraction of serum is a mixture of proteins, some of which are synthesized in liver *viz.* γ globulins. Gamma-globulins are glycoproteins, secreted by plasma cells which are derived from B-lymphocytes. Molecular weight of a gammaglobulin is about 160 kDa.

Albumins are soluble in pure water but globulins are not. Neutral salts in low concentration increase the solubility of globulins, a phenomenon called salting in. This is thought to be due to electrostatic attraction between salt ions and the charged groups on the protein, which increases the interactions with water, a polar solvent, and decreases the intermolecular attraction of proteins. Salts with divalent ions are more effective than those with monovalent ions. As the salt concentration is increased, however, salt ions compete for the water molecule of hydration of the hydrated groups of proteins, resulting in the decreased solubility and precipitation of protein out of the solution. This phenomenon is referred to as 'salting out' of protein. Ammonium sulphate is commonly used for salting out proteins.

Measurement of serum-total protein is useful in conditions relating to changes in plasma or fluid volumes, such as shock and dehydration. In these conditions, concentration of serum-total protein is elevated indicating hemoconcentration. Hemodilution is reflected as relative hypoproteinemia, which occurs with water intoxication or salt retention syndrome, during massive intravenous infusions.

Collection of Sample

Either serum or plasma may be used, but serum is preferred. A fasting specimen is not required but may be desired to decrease lipemia. Avoid hemolysis. Tightly stoppered samples are stable for 24 hours at room temperature (25-35°C), one week at 2-8°C and for 3 months at -20°C.

Methods of Estimation

The most commonly used method for total serum protein estimation in the clinical laboratory is the biuret reaction (mentioned previously in section II.9). A modification of the biuret reaction has been adapted for automated chemical analyzers. Serum proteins may also be estimated by immunochemical methods. In biuret test, proteins form a purple colored complex with cupric ions in alkaline solution. The reaction takes its name from the simple compound biuret which reacts in the same way. The intensity of the purple color is measured at 540 nm and compared with a standard serum of known protein concentration.

Requirements

1. Stock biuret reagent—Dissolve 45 grams of sodium potassium tartarate in 400 ml of 200 mmol/L NaOH. Add 15 g of copper sulphate and stir continuously. Add 5 g of potassium iodide and make up the volume to 1 liter with 200 mmol/L NaOH.
2. Working solution of biuret reagent—Dilute 200 ml of biuret stock solution to 1 liter 200 mmol/L NaOH.
3. Standard human or bovine albumin–80 g/L.
4. Dilutant saline solution–0.9% in water.

Methodology

1. Add the reagents in a tube as mentioned for various tests.

	Test sample	*Standard*	*Blank*
Serum	0.1 ml	–	–
Standard (6%)	–	0.1 ml	–
DD water	–	–	0.1 ml
Biuret reagent	5 ml	5 ml	5 ml

2. Mix well, Wait for 10 minutes and read at 540 nm.

Calculation

$$\text{Total protein in g/100 ml} = \frac{\text{Reading of test–reading of blank}}{\text{Reading of standard–reading of blank}} \times \text{concentration of std.}$$

Limitations

Hemolysed and lipemic sera interfere strongly with the measurement of proteins. Set up appropriate blank for such samples by adding 0.1 ml of serum to 5.5 ml of sodium chloride diluent.

Estimation of A : G Ratio

There are two methods for estimation of serum albumin to globulin ratio:

1. Albumins and globulins are separated by salting out with ammonium sulfate and estimated separately.
2. Total protein in serum is estimated by the biuret reaction followed by estimation of the albumin fraction. The globulin fraction is then calculated by subtracting albumin fraction from total proteins.

Estimation of serum albumin BCG method (albumin estimation)— A number of dyes bind to albumin and in this process their absorption maximum shifts, i.e. they absorb light at a wavelength different from the unbound form. This property is exploited for measuring the albumin fraction without separation from the globulin fraction. Dyes which bind specifically and with high affinity to albumin are chosen. Bromocresol green (BCG) is the most widely used dye. The unbound form is green and the bound forms blue. The intensity of the blue color produced is proportional to the total albumin present in serum. As bovine or horse albumin behave differently from human albumin in the BCG method, it is necessary to prepare standards from human serum.

Methodology

1. Add the reagents in a tube as mentioned for various tests.

	Test sample	Standard	Blank
Serum	0.1 ml	–	–
Standard (4%)	–	0.1 ml	–
DD water	–	–	0.1 ml
BCG solution	5 ml	5 ml	5 ml

2. Mix well, read *immediately* at 670 nm.

Normal values in serum.

Total protein .... 5.5-8 gm/dl
Albumin .... 3.5-5.5 gm/dl
Globulins .... 2.5-3.5 gm/dl
A : G ratio .... 1.5 to 2.5
Fibrinogen (precipitated with globulins)....... 0.2-0.4 gm/dl.

Normal values in the serum are affected by nutritional state, hepatic function, renal function, diseased and metabolic errors. Hence, variations in the plasma protein levels may signify a particular disease status.

Clinical Significance

1. Hypoproteinemia or decrease in serum protein level below the normal levels is usually due to reduced albumin levels and hence is accompanied by reduced A:G ratio.

   Some common causes of hypoproteinemia are:

   a. Renal disorders, some of which like nephrotic syndrome lead to loss of serum proteins, mainly albumin, in urine.
   b. Chronic liver disorders like cirrhosis, in which albumin synthesis is impaired.
   c. Chronic malnutrition with protein deficient diet over a prolonged period. Marasmus and Kwashiorkor.

2. Hyperproteinemia or increase in total serum protein above the normal levels, is mostly due to a rise in globulin concentration in the plasma, again with a reduced A:G ratio.

   Hyperproteinemia occurs in

   a. Chronic infections, e.g. Kala azar.
   b. Multiple myeloma—a cancer of plasma cells (the-immunoglobulin producing cells).

c. Rise in serum protein concentration is also seen in hemoconcentration, i.e. fall in water content of blood due to diarrhea and dehydration.
d. Autoimmune diseases like erythematoses, sarcidosis and rheumatoid arthritis.

Precautions

1. Serum or plasma fraction should be free of hemolysis.
2. The rate of color development varies with time and temperature of incubation, hence standard tests should be performed each time and in parallel.

LIPIDS AND LIPOPROTEINS

Lipoproteins are micelles of high molecular weight that transport non-polar lipids (triglycerides and cholesterol esters) via plasma. Each lipoprotein particle consists of an outer monolayer of protein (called apolipoprotein) and polar lipids (phospholipid and unesterified cholesterol) and an inner core of neutral lipids (triglycerides and cholesterol esters). The core neutral lipids are primarily inactive passengers whereas the apolipoproteins are mainly responsible for further metabolism and catabolism of the particle by binding to specific enzymes or transport proteins on cell membranes.

Estimation of Cholesterol

The major constituents of plasma lipids are cholesterol and triglycerides. Cholesterol is an important compound of cell membrane and precursor for the synthesis of bile salts and steroid hormones. Cholesterol is synthesized in the liver and transported in the blood mainly in the form of LDL and HDL. In blood, cholesterol is present in free as well as esterified form.Over the decades, serum cholesterol has been measured by methods employing Liebermann-Burchard reaction. The enzymatic method has become popular in recent years.

Methods for estimating total cholesterol-principles are:

1. Enzymatic method, and
2. Colorimetric methods in strong acid solvents.

Enzymatic Method

Cholesterol esters in serum are hydrolysed by cholesterol esterase. The free cholesterol is then oxidized by cholesterol oxidase (obtained from the bacterium, *Nocardia erythropolis*) to the corresponding ketone liberating hydrogen peroxide, which is then converted to water and oxygen by the enzyme peroxidase. The enzyme acts only on free cholesterol and not on the ester form, therefore cholesterol ester first needs to be converted to free cholesterol by the action of enzyme cholesterol hydrolase. Para-aminophenazone (4-aminophenazone) takes up the oxygen and together with phenol forms a pink colored quinoneimine dye, which can be measured at 515 nm.

Step 1. Cholesterol esters $\xrightarrow[\text{or ethanolic KOH}]{\text{CE. hydrolase}}$ cholesterol + fatty acids

Step 2. Cholesterol + O_2 $\xrightarrow{\text{Cholest. oxidase}}$ cholest-4-en-3-one + H_2O_2

Step 3. $2H_2O_2$ + 4 -aminophenazone $\xrightarrow[\text{+ phenol}]{\text{Peroxidase}}$ O-quinoneimine dye + $4H_2O$ (Pink)

Colorimetric Method (Liebermann–Burchard reaction), Principle

This depends on the ability of cholesterol to be converted into highly colored substances in solvents which have dehydrating, oxidizing and sulphonating properties like acetic acid in presence of sulphuric acid.

Step 1. Cholesterol (2 molecules) Oxidation $\xrightarrow{\text{dehydration}}$ Cholesta-3,5-diene (2 molecules)

Step 2. Bis cholesta–3, 5-diene (1 molecule) $\xrightarrow{\text{Sulphonation}}$ Monosulphonic acid or disulphonic acid

Sample Collection

Serum or plasma can be used. A fasting blood sample is preferred for lipid profile test. However, if cholesterol alone has to be analysed, a random sample can also be used. The specimen is stable for one week at 2–8°C and at least for 3 months at -20°C.

Requirements

1. $FeCl_3$, 0.05% in aldehyde free acetic acid
2. CH_3COOH
3. H_2SO_4
4. Stock cholesterol 100 mg in 100 ml acetic acid
5. Working cholesterol solution–1 : 25 dilution of stock in $FeCl_3$ solution.

Methodology

1. Extract total cholesterol from 0.1 ml serum by mixing thoroughly with glass rod for 15 minutes with 9.9 ml of $FeCl_3$–CH_3COOH and centrifuge at 2000 rpm for 10 minutes.
2. In 3 tubes prepare the test, standard and blank reaction mixture with $FeCl_3$–CH_3COOH.

	Test sample	*Standard*	*Blank*
Extracted supernatant	5 ml	–	–
Standard	–	0.1 ml	–
$FeCl_3$ reagent	–	4.9 ml	5 ml
H_2SO_4	3 ml	3 ml	3 ml

3. Mix well; keep in a water bath at 50–60°C for 10 minutes or 20–30 minutes at RT.
4. Cool to room temperature and read at 560 nm. Do not rinse cuvette with water.

Calculation

mg cholesterol/100 ml = Unknown/standard × 400.

Estimation of HDL Cholesterol

LDL, VLDL and chylomicrons are precipitated by polyanion in the presence of metal ions to leave HDL in solution. The cholesterol content of the supernatant is estimated by employing the procedure of total cholesterol estimation.

Methodology

1. Separate HDL cholesterol from 1 ml of serum by thoroughly mixing it with 0.1 ml of phosphotungstate reagent and 50 μl of $MgCl_2$ solution and centrifuge it for 30 minutes at 1500 g.
2. Collect the supernatant and estimate cholesterol by the total cholesterol method.

Calculation

HDL cholesterol (mmol/l) + cholesterol (mmol/l) × dilution factor (Dilution factor = 1.15)

Precautions

1. Serum is preferable to plasma and should be stored at 4°C prior to analysis, which should be carried out within 7 days.
2. Preferably, a fasting serum sample should be obtained.

Estimation of Triglycerides

Triglycerides are esters of glycerol and 3 fatty acids.

Requirements

1. n-Heptane
2. Isopropanol
3. Sodium metaperiodate—6g/litre, including 50 ml of glacial acetic acid,
4. Ammonium acetate–2 mol/liter.
5. Acetylacetone reagent: 1.5 ml of acetylacetone diluted to 200 ml with ammonium acetate (2 mol/liter). Let stand for 1 hour before using, stable for about three weeks when kept refrigerated in capped container.
6. Triolein stock standard solution, l0 g/liter of isopropanol. Triolein working stds: Dilute 2.5, 5.0 and 7.5 ml of stock std to 25 ml with isopropanol (equivalent to 100, 200, and 300 mg/dl).
7. KOH solution–6.27 mol/l

Methodology

1. Prepare the mix as follows

	Blank	*Standard*	*Unknown*
Serum	–	–	0.5 ml
Water	0.5 ml	–	–
Standard	–	0.5 ml	–
Haptane	2.0 ml	2.0 ml	2.0 ml
Isopropanol	3.5 ml	3.5 ml	3.5 ml
Sulphuric acid	1.0 ml	1.0 ml	1.0 ml

2. Mix with a vortex mixer for 60 sec and allow the phases to separate without centrifuging (extraction procedure).
3. To 0.4 ml of the heptane (upper) layer from the extraction procedure mentioned in step 2, add 2 ml of isopropanol and one drop of KOH (6.25 mol/liter).

4. Mix well with stopper and incubate at 70°C for 10 minute.
5. Add 0.2 ml of the sodium metaperiodate reagent and 1 ml of acetylacetone reagent.
6. Mix well with stopper and incubate at 70°C for 10 minute.
7. Let the mixture cool at room temperature for 3 minute.
8. Read the absorbance, while the mixture is still warm, at 425 nm.

Calculation

The standard curve is prepared by plotting the conc. of standard vs. absorbance.

Normal range

42-167mg/dl with a mean of 121 mg/dl.

Clinical Relevance and Interpretation

Serum or plasma should be obtained from fasting patients, as otherwise physiological chylomicronemia may be difficult to distinguish from an increase in VLDL. The normal range for triglycerides may be taken as 0.11 to 1.60 mmol/L upto the age of 30, with an increase at the upper limit with increasing age to 1.83 mmol/L at 50 and 2.17 mmol/l at 60. The normal range for endogenous glycerol is 0.05 to 0.18 mmol/L. Moderate increases are seen in obesity and these will often return to normal following weight reduction. Other increases may be primary or secondary. The most common secondary hypertriglyceridemia accompanies *Diabetes mellitus* and greater it is the less satisfactory the treatment. A similar increase is seen in Von Gorke's disease (Type I glycogen storage disease), alcoholism and in hypothyroidism. Increase upto 3.4 to 4.6 mmol/L occurs in the nephrotic syndrome. There is a well-recognized association between hyperuricemia and hypertriglyceridemia.

Serum triglyceride values are decreased following large doses of ascorbic acid and during the administration of halofenate, heparin, oral hypoglycemic drugs such as metformin and phenformin and oxandrolene. Therapeutic agents which are intended to reduce high levels of triglyceride include clofibrate and bezafibrate. Increases in serum triglycerides occur during estrogen administration, including oral contraceptive preparations, and following ethanol ingestion. Other drugs, which may cause hypertriglyceridemia, include the beta-blockers, thiazides and synthetic retinoids.

Estimation of LDL-Cholesterol Concentration

In specimens in which the triglyceride level does not exceed 4.5 mmol/L, the LDL cholesterol can be calculated from the following formulas.

Formula 1

LDL-cholesterol = total cholesterol-HDL-cholesterol-0.46 × triglyceride (all values are in mmol/L).

Formula 2

LDL-cholesterol = total cholesterol-HDL-cholesterol-(triglyceride/5) (all values in mg/dl, with TG < 400 mg/dl)

Normal levels of Lipid fractions:

Triglycerides	=	< 165 mg/dl
Total cholesterol	=	< 200 mg/dl
LDL cholesterol	=	< 130 mg/dl
VLDL cholesterol	=	< 40 mg/dl
HDL cholesterol	=	> 40 mg/dl

Clinical Significance

Interest in HDL-cholesterol has largely arisen from the finding that the serum concentration is a negative risk factor for coronary heart disease. The mean serum level for men lies between 1.1 and 1.2 mmol/L, with mean values for women 20 to 30% higher. The incidence for coronary heart disease increases as values fall progressively below 1.17 mmol/L and diminishes as levels increased above this figure. The risk for subjects with values of 0.91 mmol/L or less was more than 8 times than for subjects with levels of 1.68 mmol/L or greater.

Estimation of Lipoprotein

Specimens of blood should be taken after the patient is kept for one week on normal diet and in the morning after an overnight fast of at least 16 hours. Freshly separated plasma or serum should be used if possible. Heparin or EDTA is used as anticoagulant.

Lipoproteins from serum are first fractionated by ultracentrifugation and precipitation. Once the separate fractions are obtained they are quantitated on the basis of their cholesterol content.

Clinical Relavance

The hyperlipoproteinemias are disturbances of lipid transport that result from abnormalities in the synthesis or degradation of plasma lipoproteins. The elevated plasma lipoproteins can cause two life-threatening diseases: atherosclerosis and pancreatitis. Some hyperlipoproteinemias are the direct result of *primary* defects in the synthesis or degradation of lipoprotein particles. Others are *secondary* arising from a cause such as diet, use of alcohol or drugs, or disease of metabolic, hormonal, infectious or malignant etiology.

Hypolipoproteinemias

1. *Abeta lipoproteinemia.* It is a rare autosomal recessive disorder characterized by absence of lipoprotein species containing apoB. This is manifested in the total absence of LDL with consequently very low plasma levels of total cholesterol. Intestine and liver accumulate acylglycerols. Persons heterozygous for this disorder have no known clinical or biochemical abnormality but may present with hypobeta-lipoproteinemia.

   Persons homozygous for this disorder have no detectable chylomicrons, VLDL or LDL; therefore levels of triglyceride, cholesterol and phospholipids are extremely low.

2. *Primary or familial hypoalphalipoproteinemia.* It is the most common form of low HDL cholesterol. In the disease state, HDL concentrations are markedly reduced but plasma triglyceride levels are normal. It has been identified in both individuals and families.

   Tangier's disease, a form of familial HDL deficiency, is a rare autosomal recessive disorder characterized by severely reduced HDL concentration abnormal HDL composition and accumulation of cholesterol esters in the reticuloendothelial system and in other tissues. Mutations in the gene of the ATP binding cassette transporter 1 (ABC1) has been identified as the genetic basis of Tangier's disease. This gene codes for a protein that helps rid cells of excess cholesterol. Although the molecular mechanism is not yet understood, defective lipid efflux from ABC1 deficient cells presumably interferes with the formation of lipid-rich HDL.

Atherosclerosis: Atherosclerosis results from thickening of the inner layer of arterial wall by accumulated cellular material and deposits of lipids particularly. The importance of atherosclerosis is derived from the fact that it underlies most coronary artery diseases, aortic aneurysms, cerebrovascular disease and artery disease of the lower extremities.

An association exists between atherosclerosis and impaired catabolism of chylomicron remnants, IDL and LDL. Both hypercholesterolemia and hypertriglyceridemia are important risk factors for atherosclerosis. Diseases in which prolonged elevated levels of VLDL, IDL or LDL occur in the blood (e.g. *Diabetes mellitus*, hypothyroidism) are often accompanied by premature or more severe atherosclerosis. There is also an inverse relationship between plasma HDL concentration and atherosclerosis. This is because of the roles of LDL in transporting cholesterol to the tissues and of HDL acting as a scavenger of cholesterol.

Diagnosis of Hyperlipoproteinemia

A variety of diseases cause elevations in the concentration of one or more lipoprotein classes in plasma. In general, these abnormalities are detected by finding an elevated concentration of cholesterol or triglycerides in fasting plasma, a condition known as hyperlipidemia. The values for the plasma cholesterol and triglyceride levels provide information regarding the nature of the lipoprotein particle that is increased.

Usually, a simple measurement of plasma lipid levels, coupled with a clinical assessment is sufficient to classify the type of lipoprotein abnormality present. Occasionally; electrophoresis of the plasma is useful.

ELECTROLYES: CALCIUM, PHOSPHORUS, SODIUM AND POTASSIUM

ESTIMATION OF CALCIUM

Calcium is the fifth most common element and one of the most prevalent cation in the body. An average human body contains approximately 1.1 kg of calcium. Calcium is found in three main compartments: The skeleton, soft tissue and extracellular fluid. The skeleton contains 99% of body's calcium, predominantly as extracellular crystals of unknown structure with a composition approaching that of hydoxyapatite. Soft tissues and extracellular fluid contain 1% of the body's calcium. The concentration of calcium in cell cytoplasm is approximately 10^{-6} to 10^{-7} mol/L. In blood virtually all of the calcium is in the serum or plasma, which has a mean normal calcium concentration of 9.5 mg/dl (2.37 mmol/L). This is important for normal neuromuscular transmission, glandular secretion, blood coagulation and cell division. Daily dietary calcium requirement is 400-500 mg. Calcium exists in three physiological states in plasma:

a. The free or ionized form which is approximately 50%.This is the physiologically active form.
b. The protein-bound calcium (chiefly to albumin). It is approximately 40%. This binding is pH dependent. Alkalosis leads to increase in albumin binding and decrease in free calcium and conversely acidosis leads to decrease in binding and increase in free calcium. Approximately 20% of protein bound calcium in serum associates with globulin, which becomes a significant cause of increased serum calcium level in multiple myeloma.
c. The rest of plasma calcium, about 10%, is complexed with small diffusible anions including bicarbonate, lactate, phosphate and citrate.

Methods of Estimating Serum Calcium-Principle

1. *Titration*
   i. Calcium is precipitated as oxalate and then estimated by titration with permanganate.

ii. *Compleximetric titration:* calcium is titrated with inorganic compounds to which it has great affinity such as EDTA (ethylenediamine tetracetic acid) in the presence of indicators such as murexide.

2. *Colorimetric.* Calcium forms a blue complex with methyl thymol blue in alkaline solution. Sodium sulfate is added as a reducing agent to minimize fading of color. 8- hydroxyquinoline is added to avoid interference with Mg^{2+}. Cresolphthalein complexone is a dye which in alkaline medium forms a red chromophore with calcium which is measured at 570-580 nm.
3. *Absorption spectrophotometry.* It is a sensitive and specific method for estimation of calcium.
4. *Ion selective electrodes.* They measure the ionized/free calcium, which is the biologically active form.

Calcium Estimation using Calcium-O-Cresolphthalein Complexone Method—Principle

Calcium forms a purple-colored complex with ortho cresolphthalein complexone in an alkaline medium. The inclusion of HCl helps to release calcium bound to proteins and 8 hydroxy-quinoline eliminates the interference by magnesium. 2-amino, 2-methyl, 1-propanol (AMP) provides the proper alkaline medium for the color reaction. The intensity of the color is measured at 540 nm/yellow green filter.

Sample Collection

Serum is the preferred specimen. Hemolyzed and heparinized samples are unsuitable for this method. Similarly, plasma prepared using EDTA, oxalate or citrate must not be used as these preservatives cause removal of calcium by chelation. Calcium in serum is stable for 12 hours at room temperature (25-35°C), one week at 2-8°C and for a longer period up to 3 months at -20°C.

Preanalytical errors associated with estimation of serum calcium:

1. Increase in total calcium is associated with tourniquet use and venous occlusion during sampling. The tourniquet should be used briefly and should remain on the arm till sampling is complete.

2. Fist clenching should be avoided during the drawing of blood as forearm exercise leads to an increase in lactic acid and a reduction in pH which raises the level of free calcium.
3. Changes in posture can lead to fluid shifts that alter the concentration of protein and total calcium in the vascular compartment. An erect posture can cause an increase in total calcium (0.2 to 0.8 mg/dl) whereas the increase is smaller for free calcium. Hemodilution associated with recumbency accounts for mild hypocalcemia in hospitalized patients. Bedrest is associated with increased total and free calcium because of immobilization.
4. Hyperventilation and exercise lower and raise levels of free calcium respectively because of changes in blood pH.
5. Specimens should be drawn after overnight fasting as calcium levels depend on alimentary status and exhibit diurnal variation. Both ionized calcium and calcium excretion are lower during the night. Food usually increases serum calcium.
6. Hemolysis should be avoided by using a sufficiently wide bore needle as it alters free calcium values.
7. Prolonged contact with RBCs should be avoided as they can take up calcium.

Requirements

1. AMP buffer pH 10.7—Measure 37.8 ml of AMP reagent and add 150 ml of distilled water and mix. Adjust the pH to 10.7 with 6N HCl and make up to 250 ml with distilled water. Store in the refrigerator in a brown colored glass bottle. Stable for 3 weeks.
2. Color reagent—Add 15 ml conc. HCl to a 250 ml volumetric flask containing about 25 ml of distilled water. Transfer with washing 25 mg O-cresolphthalein complexone powder into it, mix to dissolve. Then add 250 mg of 8 hydroxy-quinoline and dissolve and then make up to 250 ml with distilled water. Store in a brown colored glass bottle at room temperature (25-35°C). Stable for about one month.
3. Stock calcium standard 50 mg/dl—Before weighing, dry calcium carbonate at 100°C for 2 hours. Allow to cool in a dessicator. Dissolve 625 mg of dried calcium carbonate in 50 ml of distilled water taken in a 500 ml volumetric flask and add 3.5 ml conc. HCl. Mix to dissolve and make up to 500 ml with distilled water. Store

in a brown bottle at room temperature (25-35°C). Stable for about 6 months.

Methodology

1. Add reagents, standards (S5= 5 mg/dl, S7.5 = 7.5 mg/dl, S10 = 10 mg/dl, S12.5 = 12.5 mg/dl) and test sample /QC in the order indicated into appropriately labeled tubes

	Blank	*S5*	*S7.5*	*S10*	*S12.5*	*Test*	*QC*
Distilled water (ml)	0.1	–	–	–	–	–	–
Standard (ml)	–	0.1	0.1	0.1	0.1	–	–
Test samples/QC (ml)	–	–	–	–	–	0.1	0.1
Color reagent (ml)	2.0	2.0	2.0	2.0	2.0	2.0	2.0
Mix Well							
Buffer	2.0	2.0	2.0	2.0	2.0	2.0	2.0
Mix Well							

2. Incubate at room temperature (25-35°C) for 15 minutes.
3. Set the spectrophotometer to zero using blank at 540 nm and measure the absorbance of standards, test and QC.

Calculation

$$\frac{\text{Test absorbance}}{\text{Standard absorbance}} \times 10 \text{ mg/dl} = \text{Ca mg/dl}$$

Normal values

Total serum calcium – 8.5 -10.5 mg/dl or 2.1-2.6 mmol/L.
Ionized serum calcium – 4.5-5.6 mg/dl or 1.1-1.4 mmol/L.

Clinical Relevance

a. *Hypercalcemia (>11.5-12.0 mg/dl).* Hypercalcemia occurs when the flux of calcium into the ECF is greater than the efflux of calcium out of this compartment. For example, when excessive resorption of bone mineral occurs in malignancy and then hypercalcinuria also develops.

Serum calcium is elevated in:

1. *Hyperparathyroidism:* Primary hyperparathyroidism includes those disorders of the parathyroid gland characterized by an excessive secretion of PTH that results in hypercalcemia.

2. *Vitamin D intoxication:* leading to increased intestinal absorption of calcium.
3. Secretion of PTH like hormone by malignant tumors.
4. Osteolytic disease such as multiple myeloma
5. Metastatic carcinoma of bone.
6. *Thiazide diuretics:* cause enhanced renal retention of calcium.

b. *Hypocalcemia (< 8.5 mg/di).* Hypocalcemia affects ionized calcium and is one of the causes of Tetany. It may occur in:
   1. *Hypoparathyroidism:* a primary disease of parathyroids, e.g. accidental removal of parathyroids during thyroidectomy.
   2. *In rickets and osteomalacia* due to vitamin D deficiency. The normal calcium level is maintained by secondary hyperparathyroidism. This is a consequence of low serum inorganic phosphorus
   3. In malabsorption
   4. Following an episode of acute pancreatitis when the calcium complexes with fatty acids which are released by the inflamed pancreas.
   5. Chronic renal failure.

ESTIMATION OF PHOSPHATE

The body contains about 17 mol (530 g) of phosphorus, out of which 87% is present in the bones. The rest is widely distributed both intra- and extracellularly. Plasma phosphate exists in 3 forms—approx 10% is protein-bound, 35% is complexed with sodium, calcium and magnesium and the remainder is free. Phosphate also forms high energy bonds in ATP, GTP and creatine phosphate. Inorganic phosphate ions are mostly confined to the extracellular fluid where they are part of buffer systems

Estimation of Phosphorus (Stannous Chloride Reduction Method)—Principle

Phosphorus in serum reacts with ammonium molybdate to form phosphomolybdate, which is then reduced by stannous chloride and hydrazine sulphate to molybdenum blue. The intensity of the color is measured at 640 nm.

Sample Collection

Use only clear, non-hemolysed serum separated from erythrocyte as soon as possible, as cells contain organic phosphate which can be enzymatically cleaved thereby increasing the serum concentration of phosphorus. Phosphorus in serum is stable for 12 hours at room temperature (25-35°C), one week at 2-8°C and for a longer period up to 3 months at –20°C.

Requirements

1. Trichloroacetic acid 3 g/dl.
2. Ammonium molybdate solution—Into a 100 ml volumetric flask add 70 ml of distilled water and then add slowly 3.5 ml of conc. H_2SO_4. Add 1g of ammonium molybdate. Mix well and make up to the mark with distilled water. Stable for one month at 2-8°C.
3. Hydrazine sulphate solution—Into a 100 ml volumetric flask add 70 ml of distilled water and add slowly 2.8 ml of conc. H_2SO_4 followed by 0.2 g hydrazine sulphate and 0.02g stannous chloride. Mix well and make up to the mark with distilled water. Store in a brown glass bottle. Stable for one month at 2-8°C.
4. Phosphorus standard 10 mg/dl–0.219 g anhydrous KH_2PO_4 and dissolve in distilled water and then make up to 500 ml with distilled water. Stable for one month at 2-8°C.

Methodology

1. Pipette the following into appropriately labeled tubes. Standards S1–S4.

	S1	*S2*	*S3*	*S4*	*Test*	*QC*
3 g% TCA (ml)	1.95	1.9	1.85	1.8	1.8	1.8
10 mg/dl standard (ml)	0.05	0.1	0.15	0.2	–	–
Test sample/QC (ml)	–	–	–	–	0.2	0.2

2. Mix well.
3. Leave for 5 minutes at room temperature (25 -35°C).
4. Centrifuge test and QC only for 10 minutes at 3000 rpm.

5. For color development pipette the following into labeled tubes

	Blank	S1	S2	S3	S4	Test	QC
3g/dl TCA (ml)	1.0	–	–	–	–	–	–
Diluted standard (ml)	–	1.0	1.0	1.0	1.0	–	–
Supernatant (ml)	–	–	–	–	–	1.0	1.0
Amm. molybdate (ml)	1.0	1.0	1.0	1.0	1.0	1.0	1.0
Hydrazine sulfate (ml)	1.0	1.0	1.0	1.0	1.0	1.0	1.0

6. Mix and leave for 5 minutes at room temperature (25-35°C).
7. Record absorbance at 640 nm.

Calculation.

Plot the absorbance values of standards against their respective concentrations. The measurable range with this graph is from 0.5 to 10.0 mg/dl. Plot the absorbance values of test/QC on the calibration graph and read off to the concentrations.

Normal values

Adult 0.8-1.45 mmol/L(2.5 to 5 mg/dl).
Children 1.3-1.9 mmol/L (4 to 6mg/dl).

Clinical Revalance

a. *Hyperphosphatemia:* Increased levels of serum phosphate are seen in:
   1. Renal insufficiency
   2. Hypoparathyroidism
   3. Hypervitaminosis D
b. *Hypophosphatemia:* Reduced levels of serum phosphate are seen in:
   1. Hyperparathyroidism
   2. Renal disorders of phosphate reabsorption.
   3. Rickets due to vitamin D deficiency
   4. Ingestion of antacids.

ESTIMATION OF POTASSIUM AND SODIUM

Potassium

Potassium is the principal intracellular cation. Cellular concentration is approximately 160 mmol/L, 40 times that in extracellular fluid. This high concentration is due to active transport mediated by Na-K ATPase pumps in the cell membranes. The major physiological roles of potassium are:

1. It is a major determinant of cell volume and osmolality of intracellular compartment.
2. Cofactor in various metabolic processes.
3. Its ratio of intracellular to extracellular potassium concentration is the principal determinant of membrane potential in excitable tissues.
4. Extracellular potassium greatly influences neuromuscular function.

Normal range

Plasma : 3.5-5 mmol/L.

Alterations in Serum Potassium Levels

The usual causes are impairment in cellular transfer or renal excretion.

1. Cellular transfer of potassium—The relation between extracellular and intracellular potassium is affected by acid-base balance and by hormones. Acidosis tends to increase plasma potassium by shifting potassium out of the cells and alkalosis favors the movement of potassium from ECF into the cells. Insulin and beta-adrenergic agonists, e.g. isoprenaline, promote uptake of potassium into the cells while alpha-adrenergic agonists, e.g. norepinephrine impair potassium uptake.
2. Renal excretion of potassium—Potassium filtered through the glomeruli is completely absorbed in the proximal segments. Potassium in the urine is almost completely derived from potassium secreted in the distal collecting tubules and collecting ducts.

   Causes of hyperkalemia: Clinical symptoms appear above 7.5 mmol and concentrations above 10 mmol/L are fatal.

   1. *Gastrointestinal causes:* excessive intake.
   2. *Renal causes:* Inadequate excretion may occur in:
      a. Renal failure
      b. Addison's disease—due to deficiency of aldosterone
   3. Increased shift of potassium from tissues to ECF:
      a. Acidosis, e.g. diabetic ketoacidosis
      b. Insulin deficiency
      c. Drugs such as beta-adrenergic agonists
      d. Tissue damage as in crush injuries, massive hemolysis.

Causes of Hypokalemia

1. *Gastrointestinal causes:*
   a. Inadequate intake: as in postoperative states
   b. Increased loss: as in prolonged vomiting, severe diarrhea.
2. *Renal causes:* due to excessive loss in urine:
   a. Diuretics.
   b. Excess glucocorticoids: as in Cushing's syndrome
   c. Renal tubular diseases: e.g. in renal tubular acidosis absorption of potassium may be impaired.
3. Due to increased shift of potassium from ECF to cells:
   a. Alkalosis
   b. Insulin effect: may occur in treatment of diabetic ketoacidosis with insulin.

Sodium

Sodium, the major extracellular cation, plays a role in fluid distribution among body compartments. The ingested sodium is filtered in the renal glomerulus and approximately 70% is reabsorbed in the proximal tubule. Further reabsorption occurs in the loop of Henle and less than 5% is reabsorbed distally under the influence of aldosterone.

About 65-70% of the total body sodium is in its exchangeable form. The exchangeable sodium is made up of extracellular and intracellular sodium. The intracellular sodium concentration is about 10 mmol/L and the extracellular, i.e. the plasma sodium concentration, is about 140 mmol/L. Sodium maintains the osmotic pressure of the extracellular fluid and helps in retaining water in the extracellular compartment. Along with other cations it is also involved in neuromuscular irritability, acid-base balance, maintenance of blood viscosity and resting membrane potential

Physiologically, sodium and water metabolisms are closely interrelated. Plasma sodium concentration reflects the relative proportion of total body solute and water. Being the major extracellular cation, plasma sodium concentration is the most important determinant of extracellular fluid tonicity.

The sodium content of the ECF is the primary determinant of ECF volume. The main factors regulating ECF volume are the mechanisms that control sodium balance and include the tonicity balance mechanisms mentioned above. Many of these mechanisms are closely interrelated.

Disorders of Sodium and Water Metabolism

Combined sodium and water depletion

1. Losses from gastrointestinal tract and skin: as in severe vomiting, diarrhea, sweating, burns.
2. Losses from kidney: Diuretic abuse, CRF, salt-wasting tubular disease, mineralocorticoid deficiency (Addisons's diseases).

Hyponatremia. Hyponatremia may occur in three settings:

1. Hyponatremia associated with ECF volume depletion: See causes mentioned above. In these conditions, ECF volume depletion leads to activation of ECF volume balance mechanisms. Water conservation may lead to hyponatremia
2. Hyponatremia associated with ECF volume excess and edema: In edematous states such as congestive heart failure, cirrhosis and nephrotic syndrome, although total ECF volume is increased effective volume is reduced by decreased cardiac output or sequestration of fluid outside the central circulation. Decreased glomerular filtration and increased ADH secretion limit water excretion.
3. Hyponatremia associated with normal ECF volume:
   a. Renal failure
   b. Syndrome of inappropriate ADH secretion

Hypernatremia is due to deficit of body water relative to the total body solute (sodium content). Normally increase in tonicity is controlled by the thirst mechanism and release of ADH. Hypernatremia may occur due to:

1. Loss of water alone
   a. Through skin in fever, burns, etc.
   b. *Renal:* in diabetes insipidus water loss is due to decrease in ADH secretion.
   c. Disorders of thirst mechanism.
2. Water and sodium deficits with proportionately higher losses of water. Excessive sweating, since sweat is hypotonic, proportionately higher amount of water is lost.
3. Sodium gain
   a. Excessive saline therapy
   b. Adrenal hyperfuction as in hyperaldosteronism and Cushing's syndrome.

Estimation of Potassium and Sodium

Sample Collection

Both sodium and potassium are stable in serum for several hours at 25-35°C and for 3 months at -20°C. Anticoagulants containing sodium or potassium salts are not suitable, but lithium heparin may be used as an anticoagulant. If whole blood is left unseparated for more than 3 hours or refrigerated, potassium will leak out of the red cells giving falsely increased values.

Estimation by Emission Flame Photometry—Principle

The solution under test is passed, under carefully controlled conditions, as a very fine spray in the air supply to a burner. As the solution evaporates, the salt evaporates to give neutral atoms. A small but fixed proportion of these atoms are excited to a higher energy state in the flame. As they revert back to the ground state, light of characteristic wavelengths is emitted and passes though a filter, prism or grating, onto a photosensitive device. The current thus produced is amplified and measured. The magnitude of current generated is dependent on the concentration, of say sodium, in the solution.

At low concentration, emission is directly proportional to the concentration. In direct reading instruments, the test readings are compared with those of a standard sample (of known concentration), similarly treated. In internal control instruments, the readings from the element under investigation (Na or K) are compared with the reading from an element used as internal standard (Li).

The basic components of this instrument are as follows:

1. *The Nebulizer:* which delivers a fine spray of droplets of uniform size to the flame, with a constant rate.
2. *Burner:* which should produce a steady, clear blue flame, without yellow streaks. To minimize errors, the physical form and temperature of the flame should remain constant.
3. *Wavelength selector:* it could either be a filter, a prism or diffraction grating. The respective emission wavelengths for different elements are:

Sodium (Na)	587 nm
Potassium (K)	766 nm
Lithium (Li)	671 nm
Calcium (Ca)	554 nm

Filters are less discriminating, as compared to the other two devices.

4. *Detectors:* generally photocells or selenium cells are employed to convert the electromagnetic signal into an electrical signal. Phototubes and photomultipliers are more sensitive and more expensive.
5. *Output devices:* these measure the current generated in the detector either without amplifications or after amplifying the initial current with a suitable device. In dual channel instruments, there are two separate light paths, filters, detectors and output devices, to allow for the simultaneous determination of sodium and potassium.

Requirements

1. Sodium solution 100 mmol/L—Weigh out 2.925 g dried NaCl, dissolve in about 400 ml of distilled water taken in a 500 ml volumetric flask and then make up to 500 ml with distilled water. Store in a pyrex glass bottle at 25-35°C. Stable for one year.
2. Stock potassium solution 100 mmol/L—Weigh out 0.746 g dried KCI, dissolve in about 80 ml of distilled water taken in a 100 ml volumetric flask and then make up to 100 ml with distilled water. Store in a pyrex glass bottle at 25-35°C. Stable for one year.
3. Working standards
   a. *Combined standard for sodium and potassium 140 Na^+/5K^+ mmol/L:* Dilute 14 ml of stock sodium and 5 ml of stock potassium together to 100 ml with distilled water. Store in a pyrex bottle at 25-35°C. Stable for 6 months.
   b. *Aspiration standard for sodium-1.0 mmolL:* Dilute 1.0 ml of working standard to 100 ml with distilled water. Prepare fresh each time.
   c. *Combined aspiration standard for sodium 1.4 mmol/L and potassium 0.05 mmol/L:* Dilute 1.0 ml of working standard (combined standard for Na^+/K^+ 140/5 mmol/L) to 100 ml with distilled water. Prepare fresh each time.

Methodology

1. Dilute each serum sample 1:100 with distilled water by mixing 0.1 ml sample with 9.9 ml distilled water.
2. Switch on the flame photometer. Digital display should turn on.

3. Turn the set '(full scale) F.S. coarse and fine controls' into maximum clockwise position.
4. Select appropriate filter with the help of filter selector wheel (Na^+ on the left side and K^+ on the right side).
5. Switch on the compressor and check the air pressure. Adjust it to read between 0.4 and 0.6 k g/cm^2.
6. Open the gas cylinder, remove the trapper at the rear of the flame photometer and ignite the flame.
7. Adjust the gas regulator to get a maximum height nonluminous blue flame with 10 distinct cones (5 on each side of the burner head).
8. Feed distilled water to the atomizer and wait for at least 30 seconds.
9. Adjust the 'Set Ref Coarse' and 'Fine controls' to zero digital readout for K^+ only.
10. Aspirate 1.0 mmol/L Na^+ solution. Wait at least 30 seconds and then adjust the 'Set Ref Coarse and Fine controls' to a digital read out of 100 for Na^+ only.
11. Aspirate the combined standard solution (1.4/0.05, Na^+/K^+) and wait at least for 30 seconds. Adjust 'F.S control' on Na^+ side for readout 140 and that on K^+ side for a digital readout of 50.
12. Repeat steps 9 and 10 once again. The flame photometer now stands calibrated.
13. Now feed diluted test sample/QC to the atomizer for at least 30 seconds before recording the readings for Na^+ and K^+.

Calculations

After aspirating the standard solution, the digital reading for Na^+ is adjusted to 140 and that of K^+ to 50. This is done in order to represent Na^+ and K^+ values in undiluted serum. Since the test sample/QC is diluted initially 1 : 100 and then aspirated, the initial standard values for Na^+ and K^+ (1.4 and 0.05 mmol/L) must be multiplied by 100 to represent 140 mmol/L Na^+ and 5 mmol/L K^+. In the case of K^+, in order to improve the sensitivity of the assay the digital reading for the standard is further multiplied by 10 to show a reading of 50.

In essence, the test sample/QC digital readings are compared with the standard readings for Na^+ and K^+. The digital reading appearing for Na^+ of the test sample/QC is read as mmol/L value straightaway.

On the other hand, the test sample /QC K^+ value represents 1/10th of the digital reading.

For example, digital reading for "140 Na^+ = 140 mmol/L Na^+; digital reading for 45 K^+ = 4.5 mmol/L K^+.

Precautions

1. Serum should be diluted. Concentrated samples may give erroneous results.
2. Avoid using hemolysed serum. This will cause elevated K^+ level.
3. Capillary tube of the nebulizer should be cleaned properly after use of serum, which blocks it if not properly removed by repeated washings.
4. Ideally instrument performance should be checked at routine intervals during an analytic run by running samples of known concentration.

ENZYMES

A number of enzymes are of diagnostic importance and the science of clinical enzymology is getting more and more relevant in disease processes. Initial enzymology with serum started with estimation of alkaline phosphatases in diseases related to bone and liver. Later elevation in levels of aspartate transaminase was associated with acute myocardial infarction, which also marked the initiation of diagnostic enzymology. Principally it is elevations in levels of certain enzymes, which are otherwise present in rather low levels, are of clinical importance for the clinician. Estimation of these enzyme levels in disease progress, an inference about the nature and location of pathological change associated with the disease can be made.

Broadly many factors can affect the levels of enzymes in the serum and they include:

a. Clearance of enzymes–Most of the enzymes are not excreted thorough kidney because of large molecular size, an exception to this rule is enzyme amylase, which is excreted by the kidney. An elevation in its level indicates pancreatitis.
b. Entry of enzymes into blood–This factor is governed by change in the levels of enzyme synthesis or change in cellular secretion characteristics.

Enzyme Kinetics

Enzyme kinetics deals with the factors affecting the rates of enzyme-catalyzed reactions. Enzymes are biocatalysts. Their activity depends upon pH temperature, electrolyte and substrate concentration. When all these factors are analyzed properly, it is possible to learn a great deal about the nature of the enzyme-catalyzed reaction. For example, by varying the substrate and product concentrations, it is possible to deduce the kinetic mechanism of the reaction, i.e. the order in which substrates add and products leave and whether this order is obligate or random. Such studies can establish the kinds of enzyme-substrate and enzyme-product complexes that can form. The kinetics of a reaction may indicate the way in which the activity of the enzyme is regulated *in vivo*.

Enzyme activity is calculated in terms of the number of molecules of product formed per minute in the presence of a given concentration of the particular enzyme under standard assay conditions.

$$E + S \longleftrightarrow E.S \longleftrightarrow E + P \qquad (Eq.1)$$

The above mentioned equation shows that as the reaction proceeds, substrate concentration [S] will decrease and product concentration [P] will increase.

In general, enzyme catalyzed reactions can be thought to proceed in two steps. In the first step, enzyme (E) and substrate (S) bind, reversibly to form an enzyme-substrate complex (ES). In the second step, the product (P) forms and is released from the enzyme, usually this step is irreversible, and E and P do not combine to give ES, at an appreciable rate. This process is depicted more concisely, in Eq. 1 above.

Measurement of Enzyme Activity

Enzyme unit. 1 unit of enzyme activity is that amount of enzyme which transforms one micromole of substrate into product per minute. As each lab can define its own enzyme assay conditions, test results should be interpreted in comparison with a reference (or normal) interval established and validated by the lab.

Turnover number. It is the number of substrate molecules converted to product per molecule of enzyme per minute.

Specific activity. It is the number of units of enzyme activity present/ mg of protein.

Enzyme Kinetics

The kinetics of many enzyme catalyzed reactions is described by the Michaelis-Menten equation, which is as follows:

$$V_o = \frac{V_{max}\,[S]}{K_m + [S]} \qquad (Eq2.)$$

V_o = Initial velocity of the reaction, V_{max} = Maximum velocity of reaction.

[S] = Concentration of the substrate expressed as moles/liter.

K_m = Michaelis-Menten constant for the particular enzyme.

Let us consider the reaction represented by Eq.1 again. According to the law of mass action, as the concentration of the substrate is increased the reaction will shift towards right. A stage is reached where all the enzyme molecules will get saturated with the substrate and there will be no further increase in the velocity of the reaction on adding more and more substrate. The maximum velocity is then attained and is called the V_{max}. When a graph is plotted between [S] and the velocity of the reaction a rectangular hyperbola is obtained.

K_m is defined from this curve as the concentration of the substrate in moles/liter at which the velocity of the reaction is half of maximum velocity. K_m of each enzyme is constant for a given substrate (e.g. catalase has K_m value of 25) and it is different for different substrates of the same enzyme. For example, in the following reaction, catalyzed by aspartate amino transferase (AST):

Aspartate + alpha-ketoglutarate $\longleftrightarrow$ Oxaloacetate + Glutamate

The enzyme has different K_m values for aspartate and alpha-ketoglutarate.

When two enzymes can catalyze the same reaction, e.g. hexokinase and glucokinase catalyzing phosphorylation of glucose to G-6-phosphate, the enzyme which has low K_m value will catalyze the reaction faster. The enzyme with lower K_m value has higher affinity for the substrate. In the above mentioned example, hexokinase has lower K_m value than glucokinase. The former is present in all tissues except liver while latter is present mainly in liver. Hence hexokinase can trap in whatever minimum amount of glucose enters into the cells by forming membrane impermeable glucose 6-phosphate. On the other hand glucokinase removes glucose from blood into liver when blood glucose level is high, e.g. after taking a meal.

We can rewrite the Michaelis-Menten equation to get a much more useful form of the curve called the Double Reciprocal or Lineweaver Burke Plot in the following way:

Kinetics of Enzyme Inhibition

Competitive Inhibition

Classical competitive inhibition occurs at the substrate binding site (catalytic site). Structure of the inhibitor (I) is generally analogous to that of substrate (S). It can, therefore, combine reversibly with the enzyme, forming an EI complex rather than ES complex. When both the substrate and inhibitor are present, they compete for the same binding site on the enzyme surface. Again according to the law of mass action, at a very high substrate concentration the effect of inhibitor will be negligible i.e., V_{max} is attainable at a high substrate concentration or the inhibition is surmountable or reversible. So the V_{max} in such a case remains unchanged while K_m value is raised. A classical example of competitive inhibition is inhibition by malonate of succinate dehydrogenase which catalyzes the formation of fumarate from succinate. The inhibitors which have lowest K_i value (Inhibitor constant) for an enzyme will cause the greatest degree of inhibition.

Reversible Noncompetitive Inhibition

The substrate and inhibitor bind to different sites of the enzyme and have no structural analogy. They reduce the maximum reaction velocity that can be attained but do not alter K_m value, e.g. inhibition of L-threonine dehydratase by L-isoleucine. Many other regulatory enzymes of other metabolic pathways which exhibit negative feed-back inhibition by metabolic intermediates also belong to this category.

Irreversible Noncompetitive Inhibition (Uncompetitive-inhibition)

This is seen with enzyme poisons, e.g. Iodoacetamide which inactivate-SH group of cysteine residues, and diisopropyl-fluorophosphate (DIPF) which inactivates serine residues at the active site of their respective enzymes.

Some of the enzymes whose profiles are most widely analyzed are listed below:

ALKALINE AND ACID PHOSPHATASES

Phosphatases are enzymes which catalyse the splitting of a phosphate from monophosphoric esters. They hydrolyze a variety of organic phosphate esters transferring phosphate groups from a donor substrate to an acceptor containing a hydroxyl group. The active center of these enzymes contain a serine residue. Two types are commonly estimated in serum

Alkaline phosphatases (ALP): A mixture of isoenzymes from liver, bone, intestine and placenta, has maximum enzyme activity at about pH 10.5. Serum ALP measurements are of particular interest in the investigation of hepatobiliary and bone diseases.

Acid phosphatases have maximum activity between pH 5-6.

Neutral phosphatases: Dephosphorylate Ser/Thr/Tyr residues of enzymes involved in various metabolic pathways.

Alkaline phosphatases (ALP) Alkaline phosphatases are a family of isoenzymes. They are membrane-bound glycoproteins and zinc containing metalloenzymes. They are present practically in all tissues of the body and especially high levels are present in:

i. *Intestine:* The small intestinal epithelium (I).
ii. *Liver:* The bile canalicular and sinusoidal membrane of the liver (L)
iii. *Bone:* The osteoblasts in the bone especially in infancy and childhood when there is active bone growth (B).
iv. *Kidney:* The tubular epithelium of the kidney (K).
v. The placenta and the lactating breast (P).

Sources of thc Enzyme in Serum and Urine

In serum of normal adults, most of the amount is contributed by liver, and nearly half by bone. The respective contributions of these two forms to the total activity are markedly age dependent. Intestine contributes very little amount. The contribution from the kidney is negligible whereas placenta contributes a considerable amount during pregnancy. In urine, ALP is from renal tissue. The kidneys do not clear serum ALP.

Functions

Alkaline phosphatases from different sources exhibit three types of activity

a. Hydrolytic $R-P+H-OH \rightarrow R-OH+H-P$
b. Phosphotransferase $R-P+R'-OH \rightarrow R-OH+R'-P$
c. Pyrophosphatase $R-P-P-R'+H-OH \rightarrow R-P+R'-P$

wherein R and R' are two different molecular species.

ALP acts on a large variety of physiologic and nonphysiologic substances. Though the precise natural substrate of alkaline phosphatase in the body is not known, it is associated with calcification and mineralization process in bone and probably in lipid transport in the intestine.

Estimation of Serum Alkaline Phosphatase Levels

The various methods by which ALP can be measured differ in the substrate used, the buffer type and its concentration, the temperature of incubation and in the units.

Method	*Substrate*	*Range*
Bodansky	beta-glycerophosphate	154.5 BU/dl
King and Armstrong	Phenylphosphate	4-13 KAU/dl
Bessey, Lowry and Brock	p-nitrophenylphosphate	Adult 40-125 U/l Child 40-350 U/l

Collection of Sample

Serum or heparinized plasma can be used. Stable for 7 days at 2-8°C. The activity increases if samples are left at room temperature (25-35°C) for several hours.

Estimation of Alkaline Phosphatase (p–nitrophenyl method)—Principle

Paranitrophenyl phosphate, which is colorless, is hydrolysed by alkaline phosphatase at pH 10.5 and 37°C to form free paranitrophenol, which is colored yellow. The addition of NaOH stops the enzyme activity and the final color shows maximum absorbance at 410 nm.

Requirements

1. 2-amino 2- methyl 1-propanol (AMP) buffer pH 10.5—Add 116 ml of AMP to 600 ml of distilled water. Mix and adjust the pH to 10.5 with 6 M HCl and then make up to 1 litre with distilled water. Stable for 6 months at 2-8°C.
2. Magnesium chloride (1.5 mmol/L)—Dissolve 300 mg of magnesium chloride hexahydrate in distilled water and make up to 1 litre. Stable for 6 months at room temperature (25-35°C).
3. Substrate—Dissolve 83.5 mg of disodium paranitrophenyl phosphate in 1.0 ml magnesium chloride solution. Stable for 24 hours at 2-8°C. This solution should be colorless; do not use it if the OD at 410 nm > 0.800.
4. Sodium hydroxide 0.25 M—Dissolve 10 g of NaOH in about 800 ml of distilled water and then make up to 1 litre with distilled

water. Store in a polythene bottle at room temperature (25-35° C). Stable for 6 months.

5. Stock paranitrophenol (PNP) 10.8 mmol/L—Weigh out 150 mg of PNP and dissolve in about 80 ml of NaOH (0.25 M) and then make up to 100 ml with the same NaOH solution. Store in a brown glass bottle at room temperature (25-35°C). Stable for 3 months.
6. Working PNP 54 mmol/L—Pipette 0.5 ml of the PNP stock solution into a 100 ml volumetric flask and make up to the mark with NaOH solution (0.25 M). Prepare fresh before use.

Methodology

1. Prepare standard tubes. Aliquot working pNpp solution in each tube (0.5–5 ml) and make up the volume to 5 ml of each tube with NaOH (4.5–0.5 ml). Each 0.5 ml of pNpp is equivalent to activity of 40 U /l.
2. Mix well and take absorbance at 410 nm.
3. Prepare test setup as follows:

Component	*Blank*	*Standard*	*Unknown*
AMP buffer	1.4 ml	1.4 ml	1.4 ml
-- Incubate tubes at 37°C for 5 minutes.			
Test serum	–	–	0.05 ml
Standard/control	–	0.05 ml	–
Substrate	0.1 ml	0.1 ml	0.1 ml
– Mix and incubate at 37°C for 15 minutes.			
NaOH	4 ml	4 ml	4 ml

4. Cool the tubes at RT and record absorbance at 410 nm.

Calculation

Using the standard reading plot OD_{410} as a function of units of alkaline phosphatase. Using this standard graph calculate the reading of the sample and the standard and estimate the alkaline phosphatase units present in it.

$$\text{PNP in mmol/L or ALP activity in U/L in the test sample} = \frac{\text{Test absorbance}}{\text{Std absorbance}} \times 40$$

Normal values The normal value for serum ALP in adult is 40-125 U/L. In children, the value is normally about 2-5 times greater particularly during times of active growth.

Clinical Significance

Increase in ALP activity is usually related to hepatobiliary and bone disorders. Increased ALP levels are observed in liver diseases, osteomalacia, rickets and bone disorders. Moderate elevations are sometimes noted in congestive heart failure, intestinal disease and intra-abdominal bacterial infections.

Increase in ALP

Physiological bone growth elevates ALP in serum and in the sera of growing children; enzyme activity is 1.5-2.5 times that in normal adult serum. 2-3 times increase above normal levels is seen in women in the third trimester of pregnancy.

Serum ALP measurements are of particular interest in the investigation of hepatobiliary disease and bone disease associated with increased osteoblastic activity. The response of the liver to any form of biliary tree obstruction is to synthesize more ALP in the hepatocytes adjacent to the biliary canal. There is more elevation in extrahepatic obstruction (e.g. by stone or by cancer of the head of the pancreas) than in intrahepatic obstruction. Serum enzyme activities may reach 10 to 12 times the upper limit of normal, returning to normal on surgical removal of the obstruction.

Among the bone diseases, the highest levels of serum ALP are seen in Paget's disease, 10 to 25 times the upper limit of the normal range. Moderate rises are seen in osteomalacia, rickets and Fanconi's syndrome. High enzyme levels are seen in osteogenic bone cancer.

Decrease in ALP

The value of serum ALP may decrease in anemia, scurvy, kwashiorkor, cretinism and achondroplasia.

ACID PHOSPHATASE (ACP)

The prostate after puberty has the highest concentration of ACP. Red cells, leukocytes, platelets and osteoclasts also contain the enzyme. It can be estimated by a method similar to that for estimation of ALP except that a citrate buffer at pH 5-6 is used and the incubation time is 60 minutes. The normal value is 1-5 KAU (1.8-8 U/L).

Interpretation

Measurement of ACP is mostly used to assess prognosis in prostatic carcinoma where increased levels are seen with metastasis and invasion of local pelvic tissues ACP is also useful in monitoring the treatment of prostatic cancer. Hemolysis of blood samples give rise to increased value.

AMYLASE

Amylases are a group of hydrolases that split complex carbohydrates constituted of glucose linked by alpha-1, 4-glycosidic bonds. The alpha-1, 6-linkages at branch points are not attacked by the enzyme. For straight polyglycans, maltose and some residual glucose are the end products.

Animal amylases are alpha amylases (also called endoamylases) because they attack alpha-1, 4 linkages in a random manner anywhere along the polyglycan chain. In contrast, beta amylase in plants acts only at the terminal reducing ends.

Amylases require calcium ions and are activated by chloride and bromide; pH optimum is 7.0. The molecular weight of serum amylases range from 55-60 kDa.

There are two isoenzymes:

- P type (pancreatic) and
- S type (nonpancreatic).

The loci for these enzymes lie on chromosome 1.

Sources of amylase: Normal sources of serum amylase are

- Major sources: Pancreas, salivary gland.
- Minor sources: Liver, small intestine, kidney, fallopian tube.

Amylase is the only plasma enzyme normally found in urine.

Sample Collection

The serum enzyme is quite stable; sample can be stored at 4°C for up to 8 weeks. Serum or heparinized plasma should be used since all other anticoagulants bind calcium.

Estimation of Serum Amylase

Large starch chains in helical form react with molecular iodine to form a deep blue starch-iodine complex. The endoamylolytic hydrolysis of starch is accompanied by a gradual loss of ability to bind iodine. No color forms when the chain is of 6 glucose units or less. As hydrolysis proceeds, the turbidity and viscosity characteristics of starch solution fall off very rapidly. Also, there is a gradual increase in soluble reducing materials. Any of these changes can be used to estimate amylase activity. There are three main methods for amylase estimation:

1. *Amyloclast.* These assays monitor the decrease in concentration of the starch substrate. This can be done by iodometry, turbidimetry, viscosimetry or nephelometry. In nephelometry, scattered light is measured with a detector placed at 90° from the incident beam. Turbidimetry measures the amount of transmitted light.
2. *Saccharogenic.* These assays monitor the increase in reducing sugars formed from starch. The chief reducing sugar formed from starch is maltose. In the following procedure, reduction of 3,5-dinitro salicylic acid (DNSA) is used to assess the reducing sugars formed in the reaction. The results are reported as milligrams of total reducing substances formed, expressed as "apparent glucose".
3. *Chromogen.* These assays use dye-labeled amylase substrates. These substrates are synthesized by linking amylose or amylopectin to various indicator groups like dyes, fluoresceine 4-nitrophenol.

Normal Values

Somogyi Unit: One unit of amylase activity, in 100 ml of serum is defined as that which liberates reducing substances with a reducing value equivalent to 1 mg of glucose in the course of a 30-minute reaction at 40°C, pH 7.0.

Serum	60-160 Somogyi units/dl
Urine	1500-1800 Somogyi units/24 hours.

Clinical Significance

Serum amylase measurement is used as a screening test for acute pancreatitis in patient with acute abdominal pain or back pain. Three times normal level clinches diagnosis if other causes of hyperamylasemia are ruled out.

Causes of hyperamylasemia and hyperamylasuria are:

I. *Pancreatic disease:*
   1. Acute pancreatitis
   2. Chronic ductal obstruction
   3. Pancreatic trauma
   4. Pancreatic carcinoma

II. *Non-pancreatic disorders:*
   1. Salivary gland lesions
      a. Mumps
      b. Calculus
   2. Renal insufficiency
   3. Tumor hyperamylasemia
      a. Carcinoma of the lung
      b. Carcinoma of the esophagus
      c. Breast carcinoma
      d. Ovarian carcinoma
   4. Macroamylasemia
   5. Peritonitis

Macroamylasemia

In the serum of macroamylasemia patients, macroamylases are present. They are probably complexes between amylases and other high molecular weight plasma proteins. They are not filtered in the kidneys and increases serum amylase activity by 6 to 8 folds. Amylase activity in urine is lower than normal. No clinical symptoms are, however, associated with this disorder. The differentiation of macroamylasemia from the increased serum amylase in, e.g. acute pancreatitis is most simply made by determination of the urinary amylase which will be increased if the amylase is of the usual molecular weight.

LACTATE DEHYDROGENASE (LDH)

LDH is a hydrogen transfer enzyme that catalyzes the reversible oxidation of L-lactate pyruvate with the mediation of NAD^+ as the hydrogen acceptor. The equilibrium favors the reduction of pyruvate to lactate.

LDH catalyzes the reaction as follows:

$$CH_3CHOH.COO^- + NAD^+ \underset{\text{pH } 5\text{–}7}{\overset{\text{pH } 8.8\text{–}9.8}{\rightleftharpoons}} CH_3COCOO^- + H^+$$

The pH optimum for lactate to pyruvate reaction is 8.8 to 9.8 and varies with the source of enzyme (i.e. with the predominant isoenzyme in the sample) and depends upon the temperature as well as on substrate and buffer concentrations.

The specificity of the enzyme extends from L-lactate to various related 2-hydroxy acids and 2-oxoacids, e.g. catalytic oxidation of 2-hydroxybutyrate to 2-oxobutyrate is referred to as 2-hydroxybutyrate dehydrogenase (HBD) activity.

Distribution in various tissues and serum-LDH activity is present in all cells of the body and invariably found in the cytoplasm of the cell only. Enzyme levels in various tissues are very high compared with those in the serum.

LDH activity (in U/g) varies from one tissue to another tissue. For example: Liver (145), heart (124) kidney (106), skeletal muscle (147), and erythrocytes (36 U/g hemoglobin). Thus tissue levels are almost 500-fold higher than those normally found in serum. Even a small mass of damaged tissues can increase the observed serum level of LDH to a significant extent.

LDH has a molecular weight of 134000. It is a protein composed of 4 subunits built with 2 types of protomers (H and M). It has five common isoenzymes, which may be separated by starch gel electrophoresis. The subunit compositions of the five isoenzymes are LDH 1(H4), LDH 2 (H3) LDH 3 (H) LDH 4 (HM) LDH 5 (M) Different tissues differ with respect to their specific isoenzyme pattern. In cardiac muscle, kidney, and erythocytes, the electrophoretically faster moving isoenzymes LDH 1 and LDH 2 predominate, whereas in liver and skeletal muscle the more cathodal LDH 4 and LOH 5 isoenzymes predominate. The H protomers dominate in aerobic tissues and the M protomers dominate in relatively anaerobic tissues.

The H and M polypeptides of LDH are encoded by different genes, and the two genes are expressed to different degrees in different tissues. For example, in heart muscle, the gene for the H subunit is more active than the gene for the M subunit. Thus, LDH isoenzyme 1 is the predominant form of the enzyme in cardiac muscle. The reverse is true in skeletal muscle where there is more M than H polypeptide produced, and hence, more of the isoenzyme 5 form of the enzyme.

The efficiency of conversion of pyruvate to lactate increases with the number of M chains. Therefore, the high concentration of LDH 5

(4 M subunits) in skeletal muscle rapidly converts pyruvate to lactate while the high concentration of LDH 1 (4 H subunits) in heart tissue favors conversion of pyruvate to acetyl CoA which enters the citric acid cycle.

These tissue-specific differences in LDH-isoenzymes can be readily detected by the localization of LDH activity in an agarose gel after electrophores of tissue extracts.There is, however, some recently discovered LDH isoenymes like the most extensively studied of these, LDH-C4 (LOX), which has a testis specific expression and LDG.

The various LDH isoenzymes can be separated by:

a. Electrophoresis (Agrose gel, cellulose acetate)
b. Immunoprecipatation, e.g. antisera against LDH5
c. Selective inhibitors, e.g. sodium perchlorate.
d. Ion-exchange chromatography/affinity chromatography.

Sample Collection

Serum or plasma both can be used. Hemolysis should be avoided as RBCs are rich in LDH and this may lead to unnaturally high values.

Estimation of LDH—Principle

All keto acids react with dinitrophenyl hydrazine (DNPH) to form corresponding hydrazine which is a colorless compound. The buffered substrate contains sodium pyruvate at pH 7.4. On addition of test serum, LDH converts the pyruvate into lactate in the presence of the coenzyme NADH. After some time (15 minutes) the amount of pyruvate utilized is estimated and using that the enzyme activity is calculated.

Requirements

1. Phosphate buffer, 100 mmol/L, pH 7.4
2. NADH, disodium salt—10 mg/ml in phosphate buffer.
3. Stock pyruvate solution—37.5 mmol/L. 415 mg of sodium pyruvate in 100 ml of phosphate buffer Dilute 1:50 before using phosphate buffer. 0.75 μ mol substrate per liter.
4. Sodium hydroxide, 400 mmol/L–16 g/L
5. 2,4–dinitrophenyl hydrazine reagent (DNPH)–Dissolve 200 mg in hot 1 mol/l HCL and make to 1 liter with acid.

Methodology

1. Set up the reaction tubes as follows

Component	*Test (T)*	*Control (C)*	*Blank (B)*
Substrate	1 ml	1 ml	–
Serum	0.05 ml	–	–
Phosphate buffer	–	0.15 ml	0.15 ml
– Incubate 37°C, 10 minutes.			
NADH solution	0.1 ml	–	–
– Incubate at 37°C, 15 minutes.			
DNPH solution	1 ml	1 ml	1 ml
– Incubate RT, 20 minutes			
NaOH solution	10 ml	10 ml	10 ml

2. Mix and incubate at RT for 10 minutes.
3. Record absorbance at 440 nm.

Calculation

1. Calculation of amount of pyruvate utilized
   = 0.75–[Ac–At/Ac–Ab] × 0.75 μ mol
   = 0.75 [Ac–At/Ac–Ab]
   wherein, Ac = absorbance of the control tube; At = absorbance of the test tube and Ab = absorbance of the blank tube.
2. LD activity in serum (U/l)
   = 0.75 [Ac–At/Ac–Ab] × 1/0.05 × 1000/15
   = [Ac–At/Ac–Ab] × 1000 U/l

Normal values

Reference interval for LDH = 100-190 U/l

Clinical Significance

LDH activity present in normal serum is relatively small, of the different isoenzymes LDH 2 is present in the greatest amount in normal serum.

Elevated levels are seen in:

1. a. Myocardial infarction (MI): LDH 1 rises before total LDH in patients with MI and may rise when there is no change in total LDH. Thus an increase in LDH 1 is a more sensitive indicator of MI then total LDH (sensitivity exceeds 95%). However,

measurements of LDF-I isoenzymes should be obtained only when initial CPK or CPK-NIB elevation might have been missed (after 48 hours) for they are not more sensitive than CPK-MB.

b. Values may be indirectly elevated in myocarditis but are normal in angina

2. Muscular dystrophy and other forms of muscular damage: LDH S predominates.
3. Liver diseases: Infective hepatitis, liver cell necrosis (LDH 45).
4. Blood cell dyscrasias: Pernicious anemia, hemolytic anemia (LDH 1 and 2).
5. Renal diseases: Tubular cell necrosis and tumors (LDH 1 is elevated).
6. Patient with malignant disease show increased LDF-I activity (LDH 4 and LDH 5).

Alpha hydroxybutyrate dehydrogenase (HBD) activity. An alternative to LDH isoenzymes estimation is the measurement of RBD activity and calculation of LDH/NBD ratio. LDH 1 and 2 (the two isoenzyme forms with greatest proportions of 1- monomer) are relatively more active with oxybutyrate as substrate than with pyruvate. In serum from healthy individuals, the LDH/HBD ratio varies from 1.2 to 1.6. In myocardial infarction with elevated LDH 1 and LDH 2 activity, the ratio is decreased to between 0.8 to 1.2.

CREATINE KINASE (CK)

Creatine kinase catalyzes the reversible phosphorylation of creatine by ATP.

$$\text{Creatine} + \text{ATP} \underset{\text{pH 6.7 CK;Mg}^{2+}}{\overset{\text{pH 9.0}}{\rightleftarrows}} \text{Phosphocreatine} + \text{ADP}$$

Creatine kinase activity is greatest in striated muscle, brain and heart tissues which contain some 2500, 550 and 470 U/g protein respectively. Other tissues such as kidney and diaphragm contain significantly less of activity. Liver and erythrocytes are essentially devoid of activity. CK is a dimer composed of two subunits (M and B) each with a MW of 40,000. Three different pairs of subunits can exist as:

BB (or CK 1), MB (or CK 2) and MM (or CK 3)

The CK isoenzymes are numbered CK 1, CK 2 and CK 3.
CK 1 predominates in brain, prostate, gut, lung, and bladder.
CK 2 is present in varying degrees in heart muscle
CK 3 predominates in skeletal and cardiac muscle.

All three of the isoenzymes are found in the cell cytoplasm or are associated with myofibril structure. The assessment of CK 2 (MB) isoenzyme in serum has an advantage over CK 1 and CK 3 for myocardial damage, as it is more specific for cardiac muscles.

Sample Collection

Fresh and nonhemolysed serum is used for the assay. Storage of serum leads to rapid inactivation of CK by oxidation of sulfhydryl groups at the active site of the enzyme.

Estimation of CK (Colorimetric method)—Principle

This technique measures the color given by creatine with diacetyl and alpha-napthol as a result of the following reaction

Creatine phosphate + ADP → Creatine + ATP

Creatine + Diacetyl + α- napthol → Colored complex

In the reaction, the following components are also used in the mentioned order–

1. Mg^{2+} as an activator
2. Cysteine to reactivation of sulfhydryl groups of CK
3. BaOH and $ZnSO_4$ to precipitate proteins to prevent further hydrolysis of creatinine phosphate
4. Chloromercuribenzoate for complete inactivation of CK and prevent interference in color development.

Requirements

1. Tris buffer, 100 mmol/L
2. Magnesium acetate solution, 25 mmol/L–5.4 g in 1 liter tris buffer
3. Creatine phosphate, 12 mmol/L–28 mg sodium creatine phosphate per 10 ml buffer (dilute 1: 10 before use)
4. ADP, 4 mmol/L–23 mg disodium ADP in 10 ml water
5. Cysteine, 150 mmol/L–95 mg cysteine dihydrochloride in 0.6 ml of 1 mol/L NaOH and add 3.4 ml buffer

6. p–chloromercuribenzoate, 30 mmol/L–1.07 g in 25 ml 1 mol/L NaOH, add 22 ml 1 mol/L HCl dropwise to obtain a precipitate. Dilute with 100 ml water to dissolve ppt, pH 10–10.5.
7. $ZnSO_4$ solution, 50 g/L
8. BaOH, 150 mmol/L
9. Stock alkali solution, 60 g NaOH and 128 g Na_2CO_3 in 1 liter of water.
10. α–napthol solution, 160 ml/10 ml alkali solution, prepare fresh.
11. Stock diacetyl solution, 1 ml/100 ml water, keep in brown bottle. (dilute 1:20 before use)
12. Creatine solution, 6 mmol/L–895 mg creatine hydrate in water. Dilute 1:5 before use.

Methodology

1. Setup four reaction tubes as follows and add listed component accordingly–

Component (ml)	*T*	*C*	*S*	*B*
Magnesium solution	0.2	0.2	0.2	0.2
Cysteine	0.1	0.1	0.1	0.1
Creatine phosphate	0.25	0.25	–	–
Test serum	0.1	0.1	–	–
2. Incubate at 37°C for 5 minutes				
ADP	0.25	0.25	–	–
3. Mix and incubate tube for 30 minutes, then add following				
Chloromercuribenzoate	0.5	0.5	0.5	0.5
Creatine solution	–	–	0.25	–
Water	–	–	0.35	0.6

4. Add 0.5 ml BaOH to all tubes
5. Add 0.5 ml $ZnSO_4$
6. Centrifuge 5000 rpm 15 minutes
7. Take 0.1 ml of supernatant from each tube
8. Add 2.5 ml α–napthol to it.
9. Add 0.5 ml diacetyl
10. Add 6 ml water.
11. Incubate at 37°C for 1 hour and mix every 15 minutes
12. Read absorbance at 520 nm. T–test as At; C–control as Ac, S–standard as As and B–blank as Ab.

Calculation

1. Amount of creatine in tube T, [C] = [At–Ac/As–Ab] × 1.2 × 0.25 mmol
2. Creatine kinase (CK) activity = [C] × 1000/3

Normal Values

Male	6–75 U/l
Female	6–50 U/l

Clinical Relevance

A 2-3-fold elevation of CK-3 (not CK MB) is seen in:
1. IM injection
2. Muscular diseases-muscular dystrophy
3. Hypothyroidism (CK levels are inversely proportional to thyroid activity).

SPECIFIC DIAGNOSTIC TESTS FOR INFECTIOUS AGENTS

A variety of methods are used for serological diagnosis of infectious diseases. They include immunodiffusion, immunoprecipitation, counter immunoelectrophoresis, agglutination of bacteria, hemagglutination and agglutination inhibition, particle-enhanced agglutination, complement fixation, indirect immunofluorescence (IFA), enzyme-linked immunoassay (ELISA), radioimmunoassay (RIA), neutralization of toxins or virus-activity, immunoblot (Western blot), PCR, hybridization, etc.

These techniques can be broadly divided in two categories on the basis of nature of detection:

1. *Direct pathogen detection.* These techniques include PCR, hybridization etc. which involves isolation of the causative pathogen from the site of infection or other body fluid and then its subsquent analysis. This process is more difficult as it is often difficult to get enough biological pathogen from the patient and often when the sample is easily obtainable the need to diagnosis is not there as the symptoms are prominent enough. This technique is marred by the requirement of a specialized containment region as isolation of pathogens is a biologically hazardous task.

2. *Indirect pathogen detection.* This is more widely used technique, as it does not involve isolation of the causative pathogen and can be performed easily with very little amount of body fluid. It essentially involves diagnosis using antibodies to a particular disease, which is an indirect evidence of presence of the pathogen in the body.

   In general, for the serological diagnosis of infectious diseases serum is used. Serum must be used for certain immunological techniques such as complement fixation or bacterial agglutination tests; for other tests, including some hemagglutination tests, ELISAs or immunoblots, either serum or plasma may be used.

   The following processes and techniques are used for identification of pathogen-borne diseases in the body.

Culturing

Isolation and identification of bacteria from patients aids treatment since infectious diseases caused by different bacteria have a variety of clinical courses and consequences. Susceptibility testing of isolates (i.e. establishing the minimal inhibitory concentration or MIC) can help in selection of antibiotics for therapy. Recognizing that certain species (or strains) are being isolated atypically may suggest that a disease outbreak has occurred, e.g. from contaminated hospital supplies or poor aseptic technique on the part of hospital personnel.

Steps in diagnostic isolation and identification of bacteria:

Step 1. Samples of body fluids (e.g. blood, urine, cerebrospinal fluid) are streaked/spread on culture plates and isolated colonies of bacteria (which are visible to the naked eye) appear after incubation for one to several days. Each colony consists of millions of bacterial cells. Observation of these colonies for size, texture, color, and (if grown on blood agar) hemolysis reactions, is highly important as a first step in bacterial identification. Whether the organism requires oxygen for growth is another important differentiating characteristic.

Step 2. Colonies are Gram stained and individual bacterial cells observed under the microscope.

Step 3. The bacteria are speciated using these isolated colonies. This often requires an additional 24 hours of growth

Approaches to Rapid Diagnosis Without Prior Culture

a. Bacterial DNA sequences can be amplified directly from human body fluids (the polymerase chain reaction, PCR). In this fashion, large amounts of specific genes or portions of genes can be generated and readily detected. For example, great success has been achieved in rapid diagnosis of tuberculosis.
b. Direct microscopic observation of certain clinical samples for the presence of bacteria can be helpful (e.g. detection of *M. tuberculosis* in sputum).
c. A simple approach to rapid diagnosis (as an example of antigen detection) is used in many doctor's offices for the group A *Streptococcus.* The patient's throat is swabbed and streptococcal antigen extracted directly from the swab (without prior bacteriological

culture). The bacterial antigen is detected by aggregation (agglutination) of antibody coated latex beads.

Immunological Diagnosis

a. By immunodiffusion—Bacterial agents, e.g. *Mycobacterium paratuberculosis* (Johne's disease), viral agents, e.g. bluetongue virus, bovine leukemia virus, caprine arthritis-encephalitis virus, equine infectious anemia virus (Coggins' test), epizootic hemorrhagic disease of deer, avian influenza virus, ovine progressive pneumonia; fungal agents, e.g. *Aspergillus*, *Blastomyces*, *Coccidioides*, *Histoplasma,* etc. can be detected through this simple and but less sensitive technique.
b. By ELISA–A more widely used techniques on account of simplicity, specificity and the sensitivity of the assay technique. The technique mentioned in chapter 11 describes the use of specificity of antibodies against the antigens of infectious agents and then subsequent detection of the Ag–Ab complex through enymes which increases the net sensitivity of the assay. Such assays are in wide use in detecting diseases caused by pathogens like *Salmonella*, causing typhoid; *M. tuberculosis*, causing tuberculosis; *Brucella,* causing brucellosis; HIV causing AIDS amongst many others.

TYPING FOR GENETIC ABNORMALITIES

Disorders which result due to deficiency or absence of an active enzyme involved in a metabolic pathway because of a genetic error are called as 'Metabolic Errors'. Such errors result in either of the following events-

1. Change in levels of synthesis of an important metabolite
2. Accumulation of substrate or toxic by products
3. Conversion of substrate into other, often undesirable, compounds.

Such metabolic disorders are though rare in occurrence, they are typically detected most frequently at infancy, since they are often fatal at an early age, and if untreated can cause irreversible damage to the brain. It was in early 1900s that Archibald Garrod realized that human genetic diseases are the result of deficiencies in specific enzymes.

Manifestations of these disorders differ widely and these can be prevented or mitigated if diagnosis is achieved early and appropriate treatment is instituted promptly. Several screening tests are available to detect a suspected/defective case, but the final diagnosis is only possible by estimating the enzyme levels/activity in the cultured cells from the newborn (usually fibroblast) or cultured cells from the amniotic fluid in case of unborn fetus. The latter gives the physician a prenatal diagnosis. Molecular genetic techniques are increasingly being adopted to diagnose such inheritable metabolic disease at the level of DNA or RNA, with the help of various techniques like PCR or karyotyping or FISH (mentioned in Chapter 12).

A few of the genetic errors of metabolism are discussed under:

Phenylketonuria

Phenylketonuria is the most common metabolic error (1:10,000 live births). It shows autosomal recessive pattern of inheritance. It is also referred to as 'hyperphenylalaninemia', as it is characterized by phenylalanine hydroxylase deficiency or absence, which leads to accumulation of phenylalanine because of impaired conversion of phenylalanine to tyrosine. Increase in levels of phenylalanine in blood leads to its conversion into phenylpyruvate, phenylactate and phenylacetylglutamine (the by–products), leading to severe neurotoxic symptoms (mental retardation). Accumulated phenylalanine is a competitive inhibitor of tyrosinase, the key enzyme in melanin synthesis, which leads to hypopigmentation.

$$\text{Phenylalanine} \xrightarrow[BH_4]{} \text{Phenylpyruvate} + BH_2$$

As shown above deficiency of tetrahydrobiopterin (BH_4) in the presence of normal phenylalanine hydroxylase can also lead to phenylketonuria. In this setting it is called malignant PKU. Generally phenylalanine accumulation in blood and urine and reduce tyrosine formation are direct consequences of the impaired hydroxylation. In untreated PKU and its BH_4 deficient variants, plasma concentrations of phenylalanine becomes sufficiently high [greater than 1200 μmol/L i.e. 20 mg/dl] to leads to activation of alternate pathways of metabolism, which leads to formation of the 'by-products' that are rapidly cleared by the kidney and excreted in urine.

Clinical Features

No abnormalities are apparent at birth, but untreated children with classic PKU fail to attain early developmental milestones and demonstrate progressive impairment of cerebral function. On a broader scale, the symptoms include severe mental retardation, seizures, psychotic behavior, eczema, mousy odour of urine, hypopigmentation.

Screening Tests for PKU

1. *Guthrie's bacterial inhibition test.* This test aims to detect hyperphenylalaninemia. Bacteria *Bacillus subtilis* requires phenylalanine for growth in cultures. In a minimal culture media when B-2 thienylalanine, an analogue of phenylalanine is added, the bacteria stop growing. When blood from a normal infant is added to such a media no change is noticed because the phenylalanine concentration is not adequate to reverse the effect of the analogue, whereas when blood from a patient of PKU is added bacteria proliferates because of the reversal of the effect of analogue by the accumulated metabolic products.

2. *Ferric chloride test.* To 5 ml of urine, 3-4 drops of ferric chloride solution (100 gm/l) is added. Phenylpyruvate gives green or blue color which is stable for 1-2 minutes. This nonspecific test is performed with a fresh urine sample and if positive, repeated at three months.
3. *Dinitrophenylhydrazine test (DNPH test).* To 2 ml of the urine sample equal amount of DNPH reagent is added and mixed in a test tube. Examine the mixture after 10 minutes. Appearance of a yellow precipitate implies presence of keto acids. This test complements the ferric chloride test in the diagnosis of PKU. Patients with phenylalanine levels over 16.5 mg/dl or 1 mM usually have a positive test. However, this is also a nonspecific test as it is also used in the diagnosis of Maple syrup urine disease.
4. *Prenatal diagnosis.* is possible now using DNA based tests.
5. *Blood phenylalanine level.* Estimation and activity of liver phenylalanine hydroxylase are used for definitive diagnosis.

Alkaptonuria

A rare disorder of tyrosine catabolism in which deficiency of homogenetisic acid oxidase leads to excretion of large amounts of homogenetisic acid in urine and accumulation of oxidized homogenetisic acid pigment in connective tissues, which after many years might lead to development of degenerative arthritis. Some of the features of the disorder are:

a. First disease identified as inborn error of metabolism
b. Amino acid storage disorder
c. Autosomal recessive
d. Deficiency of homogentisic acid oxidase in liver and kidney
e. Accumulation of homogentisic acid in body
f. Ochronosis (accumulation in connective tissue)

Generalized biochemical pathway:

Fumarate → Tyrosine → Homogentisic acid → Acetoacetate

Clinical Features

This disorder might go unnoticed until middle life when degenerative joint disorders develop. Prior to this time, the tendency of patient's urine to darken on standing may go unnoticed, as may slight decolorization of the ears and sclerae. These evidence are generally the earliest evidence of the disorders *viz.* urine turns dark or black on standing or on alkalinization and deposition in sclera, ears, heart, tympanic membrane and larynx.

Diagnosis

1. Dark colored urine on standing (rarely observed nowadays because of modern plumbing conditions), hence the test involves colorization of urine on alkalination.
2. Ferric chloride test gives purple black color.
3. Benedict's reagent yields a brown color.
4. Saturated silver nitrate produces an immediate black color.
5. X-rays of lumbar spine are pathognomonic showing degeneration and dense calcification of the intervertebral disc and narrowing of the intervertebral space.

Confirmatory tests. Chromatography; enzymatic/spectrophotometric determination of homogentisic acid. Patients have minimally increased concentration of homogentisic acid in blood because the kidneys rapidly filter it .

Maple Syrup Urine Disease

This is an autosomal recessive disorder in which deficiency of the enzyme branched chain α-keto acid decarboxylase leads to a block in the metabolism of branched chain amino acids (valine, leucine, isoleucine). Presenting symptoms are commonly of the CNS.

Clinical Features

Babies may be normal at birth but then they present with poor feeding, lethargy, vomiting, ataxia, convulsions and spasticity. These are due to accumulation of toxic metabolites in the brain. The characteristic feature is the smell of maple syrup in the urine due to keto acids.

Diagnosis

1. Ferric chloride test yields a greenish grey color
2. DNPH test is positive

Sickle Cell Disease

This is a disease due to point mutation in the β-chain of hemoglobin. It involves the replacement of valine for glutamic acid at 6th position of the β-chain of hemoglobin. When such hemoglobin is deoxygenated it leads to formation of a fibrous precipitate thus leading to sickling and hemolysis. With each turn of sickling and desickling the cells may then become irreversibly sickled cells, which lose potassium and have an extremely short lifespan of 20 days (Normal 120 days).

Certain factors increase the tendency for sickling. They are:

i. Acidosis
ii. Increased 2, 3 DPG
iii. Dehydration

The presence of coexisting thalassemia or HbC decreases sickling.

Diagnosis

Sickling test: A freshly drawn sample of blood is mixed with metabisulphite and a drop of this mixture is taken on a slide and covered with a cover slip. The gap between the slide and cover slip is then sealed with wax so that no atmospheric oxygen can enter. Sickling is then seen under a high power microscope.

Glucose-6-Phosphate Dehydrogenase (G6PD) Deficiency

Glucose-6-phosphate dehydrogenase is an enzyme of the hexose-monophosphate pathway. This is a pathway in which no ATP is generated but reducing equivalents such as NADPH are generated and pentose sugars are formed. G-6-P-D helps in the conversion of glucose -6- phosphate to 6-phosphogluconate, in the presence of which NADP is converted to NADPH. NADPH helps to keep glutathione in the reduced form as well as provides reducing equivalents for various synthetic pathways in the cytoplasm. The reduced glutathione in turn helps to reduce hydrogen peroxide formed as a result of oxidative injury. In the RBC, hydrogen peroxide results in the conversion of hemoglobin to methemoglobin.

G-6-P-D deficiency is an X-linked recessive disorder. In a deficiency of this enzyme, the lifespan of the RBC is decreased due to oxidative damage leading to hemolytic anemia. During oxidant stress, the RBC is unable to generate NADH in large amounts leading to hemolysis. Drugs causing hemolysis in G-6-P-D deficient individuals are grouped in three broad categories Antipyretics–antibiotics–antimalarials and they specifically include the following, besides others:

1. Sulfonamides
2. Chloroquine, primaquine
3. Phenacetin
4. p-amino salicyclic acid
5. Nalidixic acid
6. Quinine
7. Probenecid

Clinical Features

They may vary with the type of deficiency. In the A (-) variant which is a milder type, in which G-6-P-D activity is lost in older cells the person suffers from mild hemolysis, in the Mediterranean type which is a severe variant the enzyme is deficient in both the young and the old RBCs; thus the person may suffer from hemolysis even in the absence of oxidant stress.

Diagnosis

1. *Bernstein method.* Fresh blood is hemolysed and to it freshly prepared dye + NADP + G-6-P is added. The time required for the reduced hemoglobin to change to red color is noted, which may be more than 2 hours in G-6-P-D deficient individuals. Sodium nitrite and methylene blue are added to a citrated blood sample. The sodium nitrite changes Hb^{+2} to Hb^{+3}. If there is adequate NADPH in cells Hb^{+3} gets converted back to Hb^{+2} using methylene blue. Deficiency leads to a persistence of the cherry red color.

2. *Confirmatory test.* The spectrophotometric method is confirmatory. A spectrophotometer works on the same principle as a colorimeter. There are light sources that emit light in ultraviolet, infrared and visible regions. The wavelength is selected using a prism or diffraction grating. The main advantage is that the compound to be estimated need not necessarily be colored.

Galactosemia

It refers to any of three inborn deficiency of enzymes of the galactose utilisation pathways. Classical galactosemia is due to the enzyme galactose-1 phosphate uridyl transferase which is typically associated with cataract, mental retardation and cirrhosis. It is an autosomal recessive disease. The second disorder galactokinase deficiency primarily leads to cataract formation. The third and rarest is UDP-galactose 4-epimerase deficiency. In the lens, the galactose is converted to galactitol by aldol reductase leading to cataract formation.

Clinical Features

They come within days of birth. The infant shows reluctance to feed, and has vomiting, poor nutrition and failure to thrive. Jaundice, hepatomegaly may develop. Cataracts are usually not present at birth and mental retardation which develops is irreversible even after omitting milk feeds. Cause of death is usually due to *E.coli* sepsis.

Diagnosis

Demonstration of reducing sugars in the urine which is not glucose.

Confirmatory. By enzyme assays on filter discs on which blood is dried and then examined on Beutler fluorescein test visualised under UV lamp.

Inherited Disorders of Mucopolysaccharides

The mucopolysaccharidoses are a broad spectrum of disorders due to deficiency of a group of enzymes which degrade three classes of mucopolysaccharides, the dermatan, keratin and heparan sulfate. Depending on the enzyme deficiency at least eight variants of this disorder are seen.

Clinical Features

The general phenotype includes coarse facies, corneal clouding, hepatosplenomegaly, joint stiffness, hernias, dystosis multiplex and mucopolysaccharide excretion in the urine. Acidic mucopolysaccharides yield acetylhexose-amine and a hexose.

Diagnosis

This may be done by identification of metachromatic staining Reilly bodies from leucocytes and bone marrow. It may also be done by measurement of 24 hours uronic acid in urine.

1. *Alcian blue spot test* In this method, 10 ml of urine is dried on filter paper and then Alcian blue is added. After rinsing it in water, it is washed with glacial acetic acid followed by water. The urine appears as a blue spot on a white background due to increased mucopolysaccharides in the urine.
2. *Tandem mass spectroscopy:* Increasingly, tandem mass spectrometry (MS/MS) is being used for newborn screening because this laboratory testing technology substantially increases the number of metabolic disorders that can be detected from dried blood-spot specimens. Tandem mass spectroscopy allows identification of all affected infants and allows early utilization of gene therapy. The principle of mass spectroscopy is that a gaseous compound can be ionized and partially fragmented by an electron beam, and the mass/charge ratios of the resulting charged fragments can be measured. The simplest way to conceptualize a mass spectroscope is by imagining that a gas enters a small hole in the machine; its molecules are fragmented and charged by being hit by the electron beam; the resulting fragments are deflected to a different extent by an electric field depending upon their mass/charge ratios; and then the fragments are "splattered" against different portions of the far wall. The mass spectra can then be obtained by measuring where on the wall different fragments hit.

ESTIMATION OF VITAMIN C

L-ascorbic acid (Vitamin C) is a white crystalline solid that is readily soluble in water. It is a strong reducing agent and is itself reversibly oxidized to dehydroascorbic acid. The best sources of the vitamin are citrus fruits, berries, melon, tomatoes, green pepper, raw cabbage and leafy green vegetables.

Absorption of vitamin C occurs readily from the stomach. Ascorbic acid is found in higher concentration in leukocytes than in plasma due to the free diffusion of dehydroascorbic acid into cells, followed by intracellular reduction into the less diffusible ascorbate ion. Vitamin C is found in most tissues, but glandular tissues such as the pituitary, adrenal cortex, corpus luteum and thymus have the highest amounts. The retina has 20 to 30 times the plasma concentration. The half life for vitamin C in humans is only about 16 days.

Functions

1. Cofactor for protocollagen hydroxylase, the enzyme responsible for hydroxylation of prolyl and lysyl residues within nascent peptides in connective tissue proteins. Among these are collagen and related proteins which comprise intercellular material of cartilage, dentine and bone. Vitamin C functions similarly in the hydroxylation of gamma butyrobetaine to carnitine.
2. Involved in tyrosine metabolism, microsomal drug metabolism, synthesis of epinephrine and anti-inflammatory steroids by the adrenals folic acid metabolism and leukocyte functions. These functions are due to the reductive properties of L-ascorbic acid, especially on Fe (II) enzyme systems. Iron absorption as Fe (II), is also enhanced by simultaneous ingestion of the vitamin.

Requirements

The amount of vitamin C sufficient to alleviate and cure the clinical signs of scurvy is only l0 mg/d. An RDA of 60 mg is adequate to maintain near saturation of tissues in the adult male who has a body pool near 1.5 g. When this total pool falls below 300 mg, clinical symptoms of deficiency occur.

Deficiency

Scurvy: Inability to form adequate intracellular connective tissue is reflected in swollen tendon and often bleeding or bruised joints and in other areas where structurally weakened tissue cannot withstand stress.

1. Infantile scurvy also known as Barlow's disease exhibits a bayonet-rib syndrome. The gums are livid and swollen, particularly in the regions of papillae between the teeth; sometimes 'Scurvy bund" develop which may project beyond the biting surface. Cutaneous bleeding often begins on the lower thighs as perifollicular hemorrhages.
2. Petechial hemorrhages due to the rupture of capillaries often appear, therefore large spontaneous bruises (Ecchymoses) may arise almost anywhere on the body.
3. Ocular hemorrhages, drying of salivary and lacrimal glands, parotid swelling, femoral neuropathy, edema of lower extremities and psychological disturbances have also been described. Some patients develop anemia or die suddenly from heart failure.

Excess

Large doses of ascorbic acid have been considered nontoxic, except for GI symptoms. However, more serious adverse effects has been observed and suspected as potential hazards.

1. Reductive destruction of concomitantly ingested vitamin B_{12}
2. Facilitation of excessive iron absorption.
3. Reduced catabolism leading to higher requirements (dependency).
4. Increased production of oxalate favoring deposition of calcium oxalate stones in kidney and blood and uricosuria. Both benefits and hazards from high levels of vitamin C seem minimal for most people who simply excrete the excess.

Estimation of Vitamin C—Principle

1. *Vitamin C estimation using 2, 4-dinitrophenyl hydrazine*
   Ascorbic acid can be determined photometrically with 2,4-dinitrophenyl hydrazine to from the red bis-hydrazone or with 2, 4- dichlorophenol-indophenol which is reduced to a colorless form. Fluorometric and HPLC techniques have also been developed. Assessment of vitamin C status is generally done by measuring serum (plasma) and leukocyte levels of the vitamin.

Ascorbic acid in plasma is oxidized by Cu^{2+} to form dehydroascorbic acid, which reacts with acidic 2,4 DNP to form a red bis-hydrazone which is measured at 520 nm. Plasma (or serum) levels of ascorbate show a linear increase with dietary intake of the vitamin upto a level of 1.2-1.4mg/dl, beyond which urinary excretion rapidly increases. Plasma values above 0.3 mg are acceptable (Normal range-0.5-1.5 mg/dl). Those from 0.2 to 0.29 are "at risk" and those below 0.2 are an indication of deficiency. Leukocyte values of vitamin C from 0 to 7 mg/dl are suggestive of deficiency whereas values more than 15 are normal.

2. *Vitamin C estimation using folin reagent:* The method with 2, 4 -dinitrophenyl hydrazine is quite laborious and time consuming and needs a minimum of 4 hours for estimation. This method involves direct estimation of vitamin C using Folin reagent an oxidizing agent which gives blue color on reduction. It can be used for the estimation in blood without prior conversion of ascorbic acid to the dehydro form. The absorbance of the color developed is maximum at 760 nm. Variation of pH does not affect the color complex.

Requirements

1. Trichloroacetic acid
2. Folin's reagent
3. Ascorbic acid solution, 100 µg/ml

Methodology

1. To 0.2 ml serum add 0.8 ml of 10% TCA.
2. After vigorous shaking keep the tubes at RT for 5 minutes
3. Centrifuge at 3000 rpm for 5 minutes.
4. To estimate ascorbic acid, take 0.2 ml of the above extract,
5. Dilute to 2.0 ml with double distilled water.
6. Add 0.2 ml of diluted Folin reagent to the extract and mix vigorously.
7. After 10 minutes, measure the absorption of the blue color developed at 760 nm.

14

Analysis of Other Bodily Fluids

URINE

Urine is one of the most easily obtained specimens examined in the laboratory, and examination of the urine not only provides information about the functioning of the kidneys and possible abnormalities of the urinary tract, but may also lead to the diagnosis of various systemic diseases of the human body which are reflected by the presence of several substances in the urine.

Physical Examination of Urine

A simple physical examination of urine can reveal a lot about the physiological state of the body and should be performed with extreme caution.

1. *Color:* Normal, colorless to straw colored (due to urochrome).
   Deep Yellow: mild to severe dehydration, jaundice, B complex therapy (due to riboflavin).
   Red to brown: Hematuria, hemoglobinuria, myoglobinuria, porphyria (erythropetic type).
   Brown to black, Alkaptonuria, methemoglobinuria.
2. *Appearance:* Normal urine is perfectly clear and transparent when freshly voided. It may become turbid if exposed for long time due to the urea being acted upon by bacteria and converted into ammonium carbonate or due to separation of mucoproteins. Turbidity of urine indicates towards phosphate excretion in alkaline urine or presence of pus cells.

3. *Specific gravity:* Measured by urinometer (implies the capacity of kidney to concentrate urine). Normal values are 1.002–1.028. It will decrease in case of excessive water intake, *Diabetes insipidus* or chronic nephritis and increase more than 1.028 in case of severe dehydration, diabetes or adrenal insufficiency.
4. *Volume:* Normal value-700-2000 ml/day which depends upon fluid intake, solute load, loss of fluid by skin or otherwise. Deviations, polyuria—more than 3 L/day, conditions—*Diabetes mellitus*, *Diabetes insipidus*. Recovery from acute renal failure (ARF) or diuretic therapy. Oliguria—less than 500 ml/day, conditions—ARF, vomiting, fever, burns. Anuria: Less than 50 ml per 12 hours.
5. *pH:* Normal range is 4.5 to 8.5 with an average of 6 in 24 hours sample. pH 8.5 or more is found after heavy meals or proteus infection whereas pH 4.5 or less is found after heavy exercise, metabolic acidosis, chronic respiratory acidosis.

Chemical Examination

1. *Proteins:* Normal adults excrete upto 150 mg proteins/day (5 to 15 mg albumin, 50 to 70 mg Tamm Horsfall mucoproteins, a product of epithelial lining of the tubules, and the rest different plasma proteins or glycoproteins), clinically a very negligible amount. Since, the glomerulus lining is impermeable to proteins of size greater than 70 kDa, the plasma proteins are not present in the urine. So only when the glomeruli are damaged or diseased the albumin fraction starts appearing in the urine.

   Nephrotic syndrome is a clinical condition when kidney loses more than 3.5 gm proteins/day/1.73 m^2 with hypoalbuminemia, edema hyperlipidemia, lipiduria and hypercoagulability.

   Microalbuminuria is a condition characterized by urinary albumin excretion rates between 20-200 µg/min or 30-300 mg per 24 hours. This is shown to precede the overt renal disease and is an indicative of increased risk for development of diabetic nephropathy.

2. *Glucose or reducing sugars:* Normal urine has reducing sugars in the concentration of 1-1.5 g/L. Of this, glucose is 200-300 mg.

   Glycosuria is presence of glucose in the urine beyond the normal range. Renal threshold: glucose is not excreted by the kidney in amounts which are detected by the routine tests used. This level is termed the renal threshold for glucose.
3. *Ketone bodies:* Ketone bodies are 78% beta-hydroxybutyrate, 20% acetoacetic acid and 2% acetone. Normal blood levels are 0.5-1.5 mg/100 ml. Normal amounts in urine are 50 mg/day. Ketonuria is seen in diabetic associated ketoacidosis, starvation, severe vomiting, glycogen storage disorders and high fat diet.
4. *Blood:* Presence of RBC in urine is called hematuria, which is observed in nephrolithiasis (stones in the urinary tract), malignant hypertension, sickle cell anemia, coagulation abnormalities and malignancy of kidney, urinary tract, and bladder.

   Myoglobinuria is presence of myoglobin in urine and is seen in crush injuries and muscular disorders.
5. *Bilirubin:* For it estimation a freshly voided specimen is required since bilirubin is very unstable. Unconjugated bilirubin does not cross the glomerular basement membrane as it is nonpolar and water insoluble. Conjugated passes freely as it is water soluble. Bilirubin appears in urine in the cases of obstructive jaundice.
6. *Urobilinogen:* It is a colorless compound formed in the intestine by the action of gut flora on bilirubin and is reabsorbed by entero-hepatic circulation and excreted in urine. Its levels are increased in hemolytic jaundice and hepatocellular jaundice, whereas the levels decrease in broad-spectrum antibiotic therapy (by killing gut flora) and obstructive jaundice.

Microscopic Examination

1. Cells
   a. RBC- is abnormal unless it is collected by catheterization.
   b. WBC or Pus cells is abnormal and is found in UTI (urinary tract infection).
   c. Epithelial cells—Normal desquamation from urinary tract.
   d. Bacteria, if any.
2. *Crystals.* Associated with renal calculi, commonly are oxalate in acidic urine and phosphate in alkaline urine.

3. *Casts.* These are masses of agglutinated proteins in the form of cylindrical molds of tubular lumen. Many types are found but commonly seen are:
   a. *Uvaline casts:* Contain mainly proteins and no cells. Are cylindrical and transparent. Seen in pro-renal cases of acute renal failure
   b. *Cellular casts:* Casts coated with various cells like (i) RBC casts are diagnostic of acute glomerulonephritis, (ii) WBC casts are seen in chronic pyelonephritis,
   c. Epithelia casts are seen due to desquaniation of tubular epithelial cells. As the cellular casts travel the tubules they are degraded to granular and then to waxy casts, which may be seen in diseases, associated with tubular stasis.

Sample Collection

Early morning urine. This is the best urine specimen for routine analysis and is collected soon after the patient awakens. It is usually concentrated and has an acid pH. Casts and cells are poorly preserved in dilute or alkaline urine and traces of dissolved substances such as protein and sugar can be missed if the urine is very dilute.

DETECTION AND ESTIMATION TESTS ON URINE

The tests on urine can be divided into two simple categories–Qualitative and Semi-quantitative

Qualitative Tests

Appearance

Normal urine color varies from light yellow to deep amber. Urine color sometimes may vary depending upon the drink, if any, consumed by the patient. The color of urine is sometimes related to a pigment called "urochrome". The degree of color also depends on whether the specimen is concentrated or dilute. Normal urine is usually clear. If the pH is alkaline, turbidity may be observed due to the precipitation of phosphates. Such urine should be centrifuged before analysis. Turbidity due to the presence of chyle (chylomicrons) cannot be centrifuged, but requires filtration using a special cellulose filter having less than 0.1 mm diameter.

pH

Use a narrow range pH paper or a pH meter. In some clinical situations, measurements of approximate pH within $\pm$ 0.5 pH units using a narrow-range pH paper or exact pH using a pH meter may be very helpful. Normal urine pH ranges from 4.5 to 8.0.

Ketone Bodies

The three main ketone bodies are acetone, acetoacetic acid (diacetic acid) and beta-hydroxybutyric acid. Testing for ketone bodies should be done on fresh urine or the specimen kept at 4°C.

Estimation of Ketone Bodies (Rothera's Test)—*Principle*

In alkaline media (by ammonia and ammonium sulphate), freshly prepared sodium nitroprusside solution forms a purple colored compound in reaction with acetoacetic acid and acetone (α-ketones).

Note: Though β-hydroxybutyrate is also a ketone body, it does not give a positive test.

Requirements

1. *Rothera's reagent:* Dry mixture. Mix 7.5 g sodium nitroprusside with 200 g ammonium sulphate. Store in a clean amber bottle at 25-35°C. Stable for 6 months.
2. Ammonia concentrated, specific gravity 0.91.

Methodology

1. To 5 ml of urine add 1 teaspoon of Rothera's reagent.
2. Mix well and slowly add 0.5 ml of liquid ammonia slowly with the side of the tube so that it layers on the sample.
3. Observe a color after 30-60 seconds.

Result

A purple (permanganate calomel red) ring at the junction of the liquids indicates the presence of ketone bodies. The result can be graded from trace to 3+ based on the intensity of the color formed, as detailed below.

No change in color	-	Negative
Pinkish ring	-	+
Red ring	-	++
Deep purple ring	-	+++

Clinical Relevance

Ketone bodies are intermediary products of fat metabolism and their presence in the blood and then in the urine are indications that the metabolism is disordered or incomplete. This is associated with metabolic acidosis. This occurs in poorly controlled *Diabetes mellitus* and also in starvation. Normal urine does not contain methyl ketone. Weak false positive reactions may occur if the urine contains L-dopa and phenyl pyruvic acid.

Urobilinogen

Estimation of Urobilinogen (Erhlich's test)–Principle

Erhlich's reagent in conc HCl. reacts with urobilinogen to form a pink coloured aldehyde complex in chloroform.

Requirements

1. Erhlich's reagent—Dissolve 2 g of p-dimethyl aminobenzaldehyde in 100 ml of 20% HCl. Store at 25-35°C in an amber colored bottle. Stable for 3 months.
2. 10 g/dl barium chloride
3. Saturated ammonium sulphate
4. Chloroform

Methodology

1. To 12 ml of urine taken in a 25 ml or 50 ml tube add 3 ml of barium chloride followed by 3 drops of saturated ammonium sulphate.
2. Mix well. Transfer a portion of it into a glass tube.
3. Centrifuge for 5 minutes at 3500 rpm.
4. Transfer about 5 ml of the supernatant into a glass tube and add 0.5 ml of Erhlich's reagent.
5. Mix well.
6. Add 3 ml chloroform and shake well and allow to stand for 1 min.

7. Observe for any color change in the chloroform layer (bottom layer).

Result

Colorless	:	Not detected
Faint red color	:	Normal
Red or bright red	:	Positive or highly positive depending upon the intensity of color.

Clinical Relevance

Urobilinogen is normally excreted in trace and a normal urine will always show a faint red color in the chloroform layer. It is always a good practice to run a normal urine as control whenever an urobilinogen test is done. Excess urobilinogen is seen in urine in hemolytic jaundice, viral hepatitis and cirrhosis and is absent in obstructive jaundice.

Bile Pigments

Quite like bile salts, bile pigments also appear in serum during obstructive jaundice.

Estimation of Bile Pigments (Fouchet's Test)–Principle

Oxidation of bilirubin to biliverdin by $FeCl_3$ leads to development of a bluish green color.

Requirements

1. $MgSO_4$ powder
2. $BaCl_2$–10% solution in water
3. Fouchet's reagent (25 g of trichloroacetic acid 10 ml of 10% $FeCl_3$ and 90 ml water)

Methodology

1. Add a pinch of $MgSO_4$ to 10 ml of urine followed by addition of 5 ml of 10% $BaCl_2$ solution and filter.
2. $BaSO_4$ acts as absorbent for bilirubin and helps in concentrating it.
3. Dry the filter paper and add a drop or two of Fouchet's reagent at the edge of the precipitate and look for a color change.

Result

No color change in the precipitate : Negative
Appearance of a green or blue colur : Positive

SEMI-QUANTITATIVE TESTS

Proteins

Estimation of Proteins (Heat and Acetic Test)–Principle

Proteins in urine are coagulated by heat and the degree of coagulation is directly proportional to the amount of proteins present. Coagulation can be further enhanced when drops of acetic acid are added.

Requirements

1. Acetic acid

Methodology

1. Fill half the test tube with urine and adjust its pH between 4–5 using 3% acetic acid and heat the top/upper half of the sample until it boils.
2. Look for any turbidity at the upper part of the tube by comparing with the lower part of the tube.
3. If any turbidity appears, add 2 drops of 33% acetic acid. (Acidification is necessary because in alkaline medium heating may precipitate phosphates).
4. Presence of a precipitate/coagulum in the upper region is attributed to the presence of proteins (albumin), which increase on acidification. But if the precipitate is due to phosphates, it will dissolve on acidification.

Result

Observation	*Semi-quantitative estimate*
No Cloudiness	Negative
Barely visible turbidity	5 mg/100 ml
Distinct turbidity	10–30 mg/100 ml
Moderate turbidity	40–100 mg/100 ml
Heavy turbidity	200-500 mg/100 ml

Precipitation Test—Principle

Urine proteins are precipitated by sulfosalicylic acid, which gives a white precipitate, and the degree of the precipitate is proportional to the protein level.

Requirements

1. Trichloroacetic acid
2. 3% sulfosalicylic acid

Methodology

1. Add 1 ml of 3% of trichloroacetic acid or a few drops of sulfosalicylic acid solution to 5 ml of clear urine.
2. A white precipitate indicates towards the presence of proteins.

Sugars

Estimation of Sugar (Benedicts's Test)—Principle

Benedict's test is routinely performed for estimation of glucosc in urine. It is a semiquantitative test in which sugars react with Benedict's reagent (solution containing copper sulphate, sodium citrate and sodium carbonate) at alkaline pH. The reaction involves cupric hydroxide to red cupric oxide by sugars. The results are reported as 1+, 2+, etc. depending upon the color and intensity of the cuprous oxide precipitate.

Requirements

1. *Benedict's reagent.* Dissolve 17.3 g of crystalline copper sulfate in about 800 ml of distilled water, then add 100 g of sodium carbonate, mix to dissolve and finally add 175 g of sodium citrate. Mix well to dissolve and then make up to one liter with distilled water. Store in an amber colored bottle at 25-35°C. Stable for one year.

Methodology

1. To 5 ml of Benedict's reagent add 8 drops of urine.
2. Heat to boiling point for 3 minutes; keep on stand for 2 minutes
3. Note the color of precipitation formed.

Results

Observation	*Report*	*Interpretation*
Clear blue/green	Nil	–
Pale green solution	±	Trace
Cloudy green	1+	100–300 mg/100 ml
Yellow to orange ppt.	2+	300–1000 mg/100 ml
Orange to Red ppt.	3+	1-1.5 g/100 ml
Brick red ppt or clear sup.	4+	> 1.5 g/100 ml

Limitations

A number of interfering agents might interfere with Benedict's test which are present intrinsically in the urine or are added as preservatives, e.g. lactose, galactose, fructose, pentoses, thymol, formaldehyde, chloroform, lactic acid, vitamin C, dextrin, streptomycin, PAS, etc.

Blood/Hemoglobin

Estimation (Benzidine Test)—Principle

The test involves catalyses of hemoglobin by H_2O_2 to give O_2, which oxidizes benzidine to a colored derivative.

Requirements

1. H_2O_2 solution
2. Benzidine in glacial acetic acid

Methodology

1. Add 2 ml of urine and 1ml of 3 % H_2O_2 to 3 ml of fresh saturated solution of benzidine in glacial acetic acid.
2. Blue color within 10 minutes is suggestive of occult blood.

Bile Salts

These salts are observed in the detectable quantities in cases of obstructive jaundice.

Estimation (Hay'sTest)—Principle

Surface tension is lowered by presence of bile salts.

Requirements

1. Dry sulfur powder

Methodology

1. Sprinkle a little dry sulfur powder on the surface of fresh clean urine taking distilled water as control.
2. If the particles sink, bile salts are present in urine.

CEREBROSPINAL FLUID

Cerebrospinal fluid (CSF) is a clear, colorless fluid filling the ventricles and subarachnoid spaces of brain and spinal cord. CSF production is a result of the combined processes of diffusion, pinocytosis and active transfer. The majority is produced by selective dialysis of blood plasma by a specialized sponge-like structure called the 'choroid plexus' of third, lateral and fourth ventricles, but about 30% comes from other brain capillaries and seeps into the system via the extracellular fluid. The total volume of CSF is about 150 ml which remains constant and the rate of CSF production is about 550 ml per day thus, turnover rate is about 3.7 times a day. CSF is reabsorbed into the venous system by numerous microscopic arachnoid villi and larger but less common arachnoid granulations (pacchinian bodies). A blood-brain barrier exists for many blood-borne substances like bilirubin and certain drugs, so that their concentration in CSF is lower than in plasma.

Sample Collection

CSF is collected by lumbar puncture in which a fine bore needle is passed between the 3rd and 4th lumber vertebrae into the subarachnoid space with the patient lying in the lateral position and the fluid is allowed to flow automatically. The bevel of the needle should be parallel to the long axis of the spine. The whole procedure is done under strict asepsis. Only a physician or a specially trained nurse must collect the specimen. Laboratory personnel should however be present, so that the specimen is delivered to the laboratory immediately after collection. The first few drops at the fluid are discarded and the rest of the fluid is collected in sterile containers. There are specific indications and contraindications for lumbar puncture. It must be borne in mind that CSF samples must always be centrifuged prior to analysis in order to precipitate any cells, otherwise falsely high values for CSF protein will be obtained. The utmost caution must be exercised while pipetting and handling CSF samples. Glucose and protein estimations should be performed as soon as possible after drawing the CSF specimen. If testing is delayed, the specimen may be frozen at -20°C up to 3 days. Centrifuge specimens containing red blood cells or particulate matter. Do not delay testing the CSF because cells and trypanosomes are rapidly lysed once the CSF is removed from the body. Glucose will be rapidly destroyed in the absence of preservatives. The CSF specimen is generally divided into 4 aliquots for:

a. Chemistry
b. Serology and microscopy
c. Bacteriology
d. Hematology.

CSF Investigations

1. Physical analysis
   - Color
   - Turbidity
   - Coagulation
2. Cytological examination
   - Direct examination
   - Staining of the centrifuged deposit (e.g. Leishman's stain).
3. Microbiological investigations
   - Staining of centrifuged deposit (Gram stain, AFB)
   - Culturing and sensitivity.
4. Biochemical investigations
   - Total proteins (Lowry method or turbidometry)
   - Qualitative test for gammaglobulin (Pandy's test)
   - Quantitation of glucose
   - Quantitation of chloride
   - Miscellaneous like enzymes (lactate dehydrogenase, creatinine kinase), bicarbonates, urea, calcium, copper, folate, etc.

PHYSICAL ANALYSIS

1. *Pressure*
   - Normally 60-150 mm of water in recumbent position.
   - *Low opening pressure:* 10-20 cm H_2O normal-CSF leak or spinal SA obstruction.
   - *Elevated opening pressure:* More than 20 cm H_2O mass occupying lesion, diffuse cerebral inflammation.

2. *Appearance*

   Normal CSF is clear and colorless and gives no coagulum or sediment on standing.

3. *Color*

   Changes only in pathological conditions, whereas the term xanthochromia means yellow color. It has been used for the presence of other colors as well. Yellowish tinge-markedly increased protein more than 200%. Yellowish–bilirubin

   Blood may be present due to bleeding from L.P. site, pathological subarachnoid hemorrhage, ventricular hemorrhage, or neurosurgical operations. When hemolysis occurs in CSF the hemoglobin liberated is converted to bilirubin and that gives a yellow coloration to the CSF (more visible after centrifugation) called xanthochromia. Bilirubin is detected after 10 hours of subarachnoid bleeding.

4. *Turbidity*

   CSF may occasionally clot if the ratio of blood to CSF is high. Usually due to fibrin clot (e.g. tubercular meningitis a cobweb coagulum appears by keeping CSF for 12-15 hours). Turbidity can also be due to microscopic fat globules (fat embolism).

5. *Cells*

   Cell count Normal CSF should contain no more than 5 lymphocytes or monocytes/mm^3. Nature and number of cells are noted. Presence of RBCs indicate hemorrhage. Presence of WBCs predominantly polymorphs indicate bacterial meningitis. In viral infection and chronic infections, a lymphocytic response is obtained.

BIOCHEMICAL ANALYSIS

Proteins

They reach the cerebral space by endocytosis across the capillary endothelium from serum. An increase in total proteins is the commonest chemical abnormality in CSF and results from a breakdown of the brain-CSF barrier, usually as a consequence of an inflammatory reaction. Albumin is the predominant protein which is increased and globulins appear in varying amount. If the permeability of the barriers is markedly increased, fibrinogen is present which in the test tube forms a clot or coagulum.

Examination of CSF protein is done mainly to detect

- Increased blood-brain barrier permeability to plasma protein (80%)
- Increased intrathecal lgG secretion (20%).

Estimation of Protein (Turbidometry method)–Principle

Protein present in CSF is measured by precipitating the proteins with 3 g % sulfosalicylic acid and comparing the absorbance of the turbidity at 640 nm with that of protein standards.

Requirements

1. Sodium chloride diluent–Dissolve 9 g of sodium chloride and 0.5 g of sodium azide together in a final volume of one liter of distilled water in a volumetric flask. Store the solution in an amber colored bottle. Stable for one year at 25-35°C.
2. Sulfosalicylic acid 3 g/dl.

Methodology

1. Take 1 ml of test sample (or standard with various amounts of protein) and add 3 ml of sulfosalcyclic acid.
2. Mix all tubes well.
3. Leave at 25-35°C for 5 minutes.
4. Record absorbance at 640 nm; compare with the standards and estimate the amount of protein.

Normal Values

CSF protein-15-45 mg/dl

Normally the protein present in CSF is entirely albumin, but in many disease states CSF contains a mixture of albumin and globulins.

Clinical Relevance

Increase in CSF protein occurs in:

- Hemorrhage (trauma, neoplasm, ruptured aneurysm).
- Inflammation, meningitis especially bacterial (meningococcal), may be as high as 2000 mg/dl.
- Other causes like encephalitis, polio. Decrease in CSF protein occurs in children (6 months-2 years)—Pseudoturnour cerebri.

Glucose

CSF glucose concentration is 60% of the normal plasma glucose. Blood and CSF glucose equilibrate only after a lag period of 4 hours so that CSF glucose at a given time reflects blood glucose level during the past 5 housr. Equilibrated CSF glucose is definitely abnormal when it is less than 40 % of simultaneously determined blood glucose-values of 40 mg/dl are almost always abnormal.

Decreased CSF Glucose (Hypoglycorachia) Markedly decreased in pyogenic meningitis (e.g. 10-20 mg/dl); in tuberculous meningitis it is 30–50 mg/dl; in viral meningitis it is normal.

Estimation of CSF glucose (glucose oxidase method) The test is essentially performed as per the methodology already described. *(Section III; Chapter 13; page 110—Glucose Estimation in Blood).*

Normal Values of CSF

Its ionic composition is the same as that of plasma for some components and different for others. Factors which determined the access of substances from plasma to CSF are their molecular weight, protein binding and their lipid solubility. Drugs which have high protein binding coefficient enter CSF less readily. Some of the features of cerebrospinal fluid are:

Features	*Normal values*
Total volume	150 ml (30 ml within cerebral ventricles, 120 ml in SA space-85 ml in spinal part and 35 ml in cranial part)
Specific gravity	1.006–1.008
pH	7.31 -7.40 (Average value-7.33)
Normal pressure	110-130 mm Ringer's solution or 7-10 mm Hg
Color	Colorless
Transparency	Clear, free of clots
Osmolarity	292-297 mOsm/L
Cellularity	Nil or less than 5 lymphocyte or monocyte/mm^3
Glucose	50-80 mg/dl
Protein	15-50 mg/dl
Bilirubin	Nil
Na^+	138-150 mEq/L
K^+	2.7-3.9 mEq/L

Contd...

Contd...

Features	*Normal values*
Cl^-	116-122 mEq/L; HCO_3=20-24 mmol/L
A:G ratio in CSF proteins	3:1
Ratio of serum: CSF protein	200: 1.

A wide range of disorders can produce change in CSF composition and the type and extent of change is often not specified for a single pathological condition.

A. Cerebral dysfunction
1. Infections: Meningitis (purulent, aseptic)
   - Encephalitis
   - Neurosyphilis (acute)
   - TB meningitis
2. Cerebrovascular disorders
   - Stroke
   - Subarachnoid haemoritiage
   - Venous thrombosis
3. Dementia and degenerative disorders
   - Alzheimer's disease
   - Huntington's disease
   - Wilson's disease
4. Neoplastic disorders
   - Meningial carcinomatosis
   - Secondary deposits
5. Metabolic disorders
   - Hepatic encephalopathy
   - Uremic encephalopathy
6. Demyelinating disorders
   - Multiple sclerosis
7. Autoimmune sarcoid
8. Other disorders like normal pressure hydrocephalus or pseudo-tumor cerebri.

B. Cranial nerve dysfunction
1. Miller-Fischer variant of GBS
2. Lyme's disease

C. Motor dysfunction
   1. CNS: Parkinson's disease or neurosyphilis (paretic) tetanus
   2. Motor neuron:
      – Amyotrophic lateral sclerosis (ALS)
      – Guillain-Barre syndrome (CBS)

D. Cerebellar: Cerebellitis

E. Sensory dysfunction: Neuropathy: Diabetic or CIDP (Chronic inflammatory demyelinating polyradiculopathy) trauma.

F. Head injury

G. Fractured vertebrae.

AMNIOTIC FLUID

Amniotic fluid is the content of amniotic sac that surrounds the embryo and fetus. Throughout the intrauterine life the fetus lives within this fluid compartment. It provides a non-restricting environment in which the fetus can readily move. It cushions the fetus against possible trauma and maintains a constant temperature. Amniotic fluid has both maternal and fetal origin. In the early stages of development, most of the fluid is derived from the maternal tissue and in later stages it is more of fetal origin. The maternal contribution consists of diffusion from: (1) decidua parietalis across amniochorionic membrane and (2) Blood in the intervillous space of the placenta. The fetus contributes to the amniotic fluid by (a) fetal urine (b) secretions from tracheobronchial tree and (c) ingestion by fetus and absorption in intestines. Any alteration in this homeostasis affects the volume of the amniotic fluid.

Amniotic fluid is usually obtained at 14 to 16 weeks of gestation or even earlier with the help of ultrasound guided tissue collection techniques.

Use

A. *Diagnostic:* In early month of pregnancy for detecting
   a. Neural tube defect,
   b. Inborn error of metabolism.
   c. Karyotyping and other chromosomal disorders like Down's syndrome.

   In later month of pregnancy.
   a. Fetal maturation.
   b. Fetal distress.
   c. Rh incompatibility

B. Management of Rh incompatibility of mother and fetus by predicting the severity of hemolytic disease in the fetus.

Normal Composition

The serum osmolality and sodium, urea and creatinine content of maternal serum and amniotic fluid are not significantly different. This suggests that amniotic fluid is an ultrafiltrate of maternal serum.

In the first half of the pregnancy amniotic fluid appears to maintain the extracellular fluid chemistry of the fetus. In the second half-amniotic fluid reflects the development of fetal renal function and by virtue of cells shed the morphological development of skin and mucous membranes.

Some typical features of the amniotic fluid are:

Features	*Normal values*
Volume	800 ml (300-1400 ml) at term
Specific gravity	1.008
Color	Straw color
pH	72
Creatinine	2.2 mg/dl
Glucose	32 mg/dl
Urea	l8 mg/dl
Chloride	103 mg/dl
Sodium	126 mmol/L
Potassium	4.3 mmol/L
Total protein	0.3 g/dl
Total bilirubin	0.04 mg/dl
Sodium	126 mmol/L
L/S	> 2
Uric acid	10.4 mg/dl

Examination of Amniotic Fluid

1. *Gross examination*: Appearance

Color	*Condition*
Pale straw	Normal
Green	Fetal distress (Due to meconium stain)
Golden	Rh incompatibility. (Due to bile stain)
Dark brown (tobacco juice)	Intrauterine fetal death
Brown	Severe hemolysis
Red	Fresh hemorrhage

2. *Cytological studies*: Cells present in the amniotic fluid originate in the fetus and these cells can be used for karyotyping, sex determination and cell culture for enzymatic studies.
3. *Biochemical studies*:
   a. *Bilirubin:* Hemolytic disease of newborn is most commonly caused by Rh incompatibility—mother being Rh (–) and the

fetus Rh (+). In these cases, the first fetus with Rh incompatibility sensitizes the mother and the subsequent pregnancies with Rh incompatibility are affected. Antibodies from mother cross the placenta and cause hemolysis in fetus and thus hyperbilirubinemia. Estimation of bilirubin in the amniotic fluid gives a good estimate of the severity of hemolytic disease. This hemolysis and hyperbilirubinemia can cause a spectrum of effect from mild jaundice in newborn to hydrops fetalis (fetal death). In normal pregnancy, bilirubin decreases progressively and is undetectable by the 36th week. Bilirubin can be estimated directly by taking the optical density at 450 nm (by the spectrophotometer or colorimetric methods).

b. *Phospholipids:* Lecithin is the most abundant phospholipid in the amniotic fluid. The lecithin to sphingomyelin (L/S) ratio is used to assess fetal lung maturity. If the L/S ratio is more than 2, there is very little risk of respiratory distress syndrome, i.e. the fetal lungs are mature, if the L/S ratio is less than 2 there is a significant risk of RDS. L/S ratio can be measured by the foam stability test or by thin layer chromatography. In diabetic mothers, phosphatidylglycerol is used in conjunction with L/S ratio to assess fetal maturity.

   Estimation of phospholipids (foam stability test)—Principle: This test involves the shaking of a sample of amniotic fluid with alcohol. Phospholipids act as foaming agent while alcohol inhibits bubble formation. If the bubbles persist after shaking it means phospholipids are present in large quantities and the L/S ratio is predicted to be more than 2.

   Methodology:

   1. Take 4 tests tubes.
   2. Take 1ml each of different dilutions of amniotic fluid (1:1, 1:2, 1:3 and 1:4) with normal saline.
   3. Add 1 ml of 95% ethanol to each tube.
   4. Shake for 15 secs.
   5. Note the presence of foam in the tubes after 15 minutes.

c. *Hormones:* Amniotic fluid contains different hormones like estrogen, hCG, LH (leuteinising hormone), prolactin and cortisol. The levels of these hormones in the amniotic fluid indicate fetal maturity. For example, cortisol level in amniotic fluid at term reaches 72.4 ng/ml. It has been observed that cortisol level higher than 60 ng/ml is generally associated with L/S ratio greater than 2.0 and values less than 40 ng/ml is associated with L/S ratio of less than 1.5.

d. *Creatinine*: Creatinine concentration rises towards term. A concentration of 1 mg/dl or less indicates prematurity and values of 1.5 mg/dl or above indicate maturity of the fetus.

e. *Alpha-fetoprotein*: Alpha-fetoprotein (AFP) is a protein produced by the fetal liver. The function of the protein is unknown. It is present in high concentration in fetal blood and in lower concentration in fetal urine. AFP is present in amniotic fluid which is composed primarily of fetal urine. Amniotic fluid AFP (AFAFP) may be elevated in open fetal body wall defects, most commonly open neural tube defects (NTD) and open ventral wall defects, due to transudation from exposed fetal vessels and tissue. AFAFP is elevated in congenital nephrosis from increased glomerular filtration of this relatively small protein. In cases with elevated AFAFP, the risk for an open NTD or other fetal abnormality depends on the degree of elevation in the AFAFP MoM (multiple of the median), the results of amniotic fluid acetylcholinesterase testing and other significant risk factors.

f. *Prenatal detection of familial metabolic disorders*: The cells present in the amniotic fluid can be used to diagnose metabolic disorders like galactosemia, Pompe's disease, Tay-Sach disease, etc.

g. *Prenatal detection of chromosomal disorders:* Amniotic fluid cells can be cultured and karyotyped to study chromosomal disorders, e.g. Down's syndrome.

Part—IV:

Tests for Specific Organ Functions

15 Tests for Specific Organ Functions

LIVER

The liver plays a key role in a variety of metabolic, synthetic and excretory functions. Abnormalities in liver function tests reflect not only damage to the hepatic cell, but also give clues to the site, extent and nature of the pathological process. "Liver function tests" is a misnomer for a host of lab tests that identify liver injury. The routine LFTs include:

1. Serum bilirubin (Total and conjugated), urinary bilirubin, urinary urobilinogen
2. Serum enzymes:
   a. Alanine aminotransferase (ALT)/SGPT
   b. Aspartate aminotransferase (AST)/SGOT
   c. Alkaline phosphatase
   d. Gamma glutamyl transferase (transpeptidase)
   e. 5' nucleotidase
3. Serum albumin and total proteins
4. Prothrombin time, clotting time

Specialized tests include those for viral markers (e.g. HbsAg), immunological markers and inherited metabolic disorders of the liver (e.g. Wilson's disease).

Jaundice is the commonest mode of presentation in patients with liver diseases. Jaundice is a clinicopathological condition characterized by yellowish discoloration of the skin and mucous membrane, sc palate and nailbeds caused by deposition of bilirubin in the tissues, when the level of which is usually more than 2 to 2.5 mg/dl in the serum. The normal level is 0.3-1 mg/dl. Hyperbilirubinemia occurs when levels are over l mg/dl. Bilirubin is formed by the reticulo-endothelial cells of the liver from ferroporphyrin ring obtained mainly from Hb of erythrocytes and also from myoglobin and iron containing enzymes. Bilirubin exists in blood in either conjugated or unconjugated forms. Normally, most of the bilirubin found in blood is of the unconjugated form. Conjugation of bilirubin occurs in the liver and the conjugated form, which is water soluble, can pass through in the urine whereas the unconjugated form cannot. Bilirubin is excreted in the bile mainly in the form of bilirubin diglucuronide. In the intestine, it is converted to urobilinogen by the action of bacterial flora. Some of the urobilinogen gets reabsorbed and undergoes enterohepatic circulation as well as excretion by the kidneys. The rest is excreted in the faeces as stercobilinogen. Urobilinogen gets oxidised to urobilin by atmospheric oxygen after excretion in the urine and so also is stercobilinogen oxidized to stercobilin.

Jaundice can further be divided into 3 types:

a. *Hemolytic.* Due to excessive hemolysis; usually results in a predominant increase in unconjugated bilirubin; also termed retention hyperbilirubinemia or alcoholic jaundice, e.g. sickle cell anemia, thalassemia, drug induced jaundice, resorption of a hematoma.

b. *Hepatocellular.* Due to damage to hepatocytes; results in increases in both the direct and indirect fractions; depending on the nature and extent of the disorder the predominant increase may be in either the unconjugated farm (e.g. neonatal jaundice—levels over 20 mg/dl cause kernicterus, Gilbert's disease, the Crigler-Najjar syndromes) or the conjugated form (e.g. viral hepatitis, drugs, alcohol, sepsis, congestive cardiac failure, Dubin-Johnson and Rotor syndromes)

c. *Obstructive.* Due to obstruction of flow of bile (e.g. stone, stricture or tumor in the bile tract).

This classification of jaundice is not strictly mutually exclusive as any given patient may have features of more than one type of jaundice depending on the nature and extent of disease(s).

DETERMINATION OF SERUM BILIRUBIN

Sample collection Serum or plasma can be used. Avoid hemolysis as it results in falsely low values. A brown bottle is used to collect the specimen to prevent exposure to light. Morning fasting specimen is ideal to avoid lipemia. As usual, universal precautions have to be taken to avoid the risk of biohazards.

Estimation of Serum Bilirubin (Van den Bergh Reaction)—*Principle*

Bilirubin is demonstrated qualitatively and quantitatively by means of diazo reagent. Diazotized sulphanilic acid (sulphanilic acid treated with a mixture of sodium nitrite and HCl) in the presence of bilirubin forms a red compound azobilirubin which is measured colorimetrically.

When the reaction is carried out in aqueous medium, the water soluble conjugated bilirubin reacts to give the so-called direct Van den Bergh reaction. When the reaction is carried out in methanol, the intramolecular hydrogen bonds of unconjugated bilirubin are broken, thus both conjugated and unconjugated pigments react giving a measure of total bilirubin. Hence, the unconjugated (indirect) fraction is obtained by subtracting the conjugated value from total bilirubin.

Requirements

1. Diazo reagent–Solution A, 1 gm sulphanilic acid in 15 ml of conc. HCl. With volume made upto 1 liter; Solution B, 0.5 gm sodium nitrate in 1 liter distilled water. Mix 0.3 ml of solution B to 10 ml of solution A.
2. Methanol
3. Standard bilirubin solution–200 µmol in chloroform.

Methodology

1. Mark tubes 1 for total and 2 for conjugated bilirubin.
2. Take 7 tubes T1, T2, C1, C2, B1, B2, and S. Add 2 ml distilled water in the blank tubes (B1 and B2) and 1.8 ml distilled water in others and.
3. Take 0.2 ml serum in the tests (T1 and T2) and controls (C1 and C2).
4. Add 0.5 ml diazo reagent to the tests and 0.5 ml diazo blank to the controls and blanks.
5. Add 2.5 ml methanol to T1, C1 and B1 and 2.5 ml water to T2, C2 and B2. (A secondary standard is used and nothing extra has to be added to the S tube).

6. Read absorbance at 540 nm-within one minute for conjugated bilirubin (T2, C2 and B2), and after 30 minutes for total (T1, C1 and B1).

Estimation of Bilirubin (Spectrophotometric Determination)

Absorbance is read directly as bilirubin absorbs at 454 nm. This method is usually adopted for neonates.

Estimation of Bilirubin in Urine (Fouchet's Test)

Refer Section III; Chapter 14—Analysis of Other Bodily Fluids; Page no. 181—Urine, under Heading Bile Pigment, page no. 187.

Normal Values

0.3–1 mg/dl

Hyperbilirubinemia	> 1 mg/dl
Jaundice manifested	> 2-2.5 mg/dl

DETERMINATION OF SERUM UROBILINOGEN

Estimation of Urobilinogen (Ehrlich's Aldehyde Test)—Principle

p-dimethylamino benzaldehyde in a strongly acidic solution gives a red color with urobilinogen. This reaction depends upon the central methane group in urobilinogen.

Estimation of Urobilinogen (Hay's Test)

Principle and Methodology

1. Take 2 test tubes one containing distilled water (control) and the other containing urine having bile salts (test).
2. Sprinkle a few particles of sulfur in both tubes.
3. Sulfur particles will float in control tube while they will settle down in test tube because the bile salts have lowered the surface tension.

DETERMINATION OF TRANSAMINASES

The two transaminases of diagnostic importance are:

1. Serum glutamic oxaloacetate transaminase (SGOT) or aspartate amino transferase (AST), and
2. Serum glutamic pyruvate transaminase (SGPT) or alanine amino transferase (ALT).

The following reactions are catalyzed by these enzymes.

A. SGOT

$$\text{Glutamic acid + Oxaloacetic acid} \xrightarrow{\text{AST (SGOT)}} \alpha\text{-ketoglutaric acid + Aspartic acid}$$

B. SGPT

$$\text{Glutamic acid + Pyruvic acid} \xrightarrow{\text{ALT (SGPT)}} \text{A Acid + Alanine}$$

For both reactions, pyridoxal-5'-phosphate is the cofactor.

While AST is found in every tissue of the body, including red blood cells, and is particularly high in the cardiac muscle, ALT is present in moderately high concentration in liver and low in cardiac, skeletal muscle and other tissues. Both AST and ALT measurements are useful in the diagnosis and monitoring of patients with hepatocellular disease.

Estimation of Transaminases (Colorimetric End-point Method)—*Principle*

Transamination is the process in which an amino group is transferred from amino acid to an α-keto acid. The enzymes responsible for transamination are called transaminases. The substrates in the reaction are α-ketoglutaric acid (α KG) plus L-aspartate for AST, and a KG plus L-alanine for ALT. The products formed by enzyme action are glutamate and oxaloacetate for AST and glutamate and pyruvate for ALT. Addition of 2,4, dinitrophenylhydrazine results in the formation of hydrazone complex with the ketoacids. A red color is produced on the addition of sodium hydroxide. The intensity of color is related to enzymatic activity.

Sample Collection

Serum or EDTA/heparinized plasma can be used in this assay. Transaminases are stable in serum for 6 hours at 25-35°C, 7 days at 2-8°C and for one month when stored at -20°C.

Requirements

1. Phosphate buffer, pH 7.4
2. AST substrate—Dissolve 2.66 g DL—aspartic acid and 30 mg α-ketoglutarate in 20.5 ml of 1 M NaOH. Adjust the pH to 7.4 by adding 1 M NaOH drop wise while stirring. Make up to 100 ml with phosphate buffer. Add 1 ml of chloroform as preservative. Stable for 2 months when stored at 2-8° C. Discard if it becomes turbid.
3. ALT substrate—Dissolve 1.78 g DL-alanine and 30 mg α-ketoglutarate in 20 ml of phosphate buffer containing 1.25 ml of 0.4 M NaOH. Make up to 100 ml with buffer and adjust to pH 7.4 if necessary. Add 1 ml chloroform as preservative. Stable for 2 months when stored at 2-8°C. Discard if it becomes turbid.
4. Pyruvate standard 2 mmol/ml—Dissolve 220 mg sodium pyruvate in phosphate buffer and make up to 100 ml. Dilute 10 ml of this solution to 100 ml with phosphate buffer to obtain the working standard containing 2 mmol pyruvate per ml.
5. Color reagent—Dissolve 200 mg 2,4 dinitrophenylhydrazine (2,4-DNPH) in hot 1M HCl and make up to 1 liter with 1M HCl. Stable for 6 months when stored at 2 -8°C.
6. 0.4 M sodium hydroxide—Dissolve 16 g sodium hydroxide in about 800 ml of distilled water and make up to 1 liter with distilled water. Store in a polyethylene container at 25-35°C. Stable for 6 months.

Methodology

1. In 4 test tubes setup the reaction as below:

	Test blank	*Control blank*	*Test*	*Standard*
AST substrate (ml)	0.5	0.5	0.5	0.5
Test sample/QC (ml)	–	–	0.1	0.1

2. Mix and incubate at 37 °C in a water bath for 1 hour the add DNPH solution

2,4 DNPH (ml)	0.5	0.5	0.5	0.5
Mix and remove the tubes from the water bath, followed by addition of test sample				
Test sample/QC (ml)	0.1	0.1	–	–

3. Mix and leave the tubes for 20 minutes at room temperature (25-35°C)

0.4M NaOH (ml)	5.0	5.0	5.0	5.0

4. Mix and leave the tubes for 5 minutes at room temperature (25-35°C)
5. Set the spectrophotometer to zero and measure absorbance at 510 nm.

Note: In Step 2 the incubation time is 1 hour for AST (SGOT) and 30 minutes for ALT (SGPT). Rest of the protocol is same for both the methods using their respective substrates.

Calculation

Activity of the enzymes is determined in terms of U/L, i.e. micromoles of product formed or micromoles of substrate used up per minute per liter, i.e. mmoles of pyruvate/min/l. In the measurement of both serum AST and ALT, only pyruvate is used as the standard. Theoretically speaking, oxaloacetate should be used as the standard for AST assay and pyruvate as the standard for ALT assay. Oxaloacetate formed in the AST assay is unstable and immediately gets converted into pyruvate; hence the use of pyruvate standard for AST assay.

Using a standard graph plotted using various concentrations of pyruvate (0.1 to 0.4 μmol) as a function of spectrophotometric absorbance, the amount of pyruvate present in the test sample can be estimated. The volume of pyruvate should be 0.6 ml and the reaction should be carried out as described in the protocol.

Normal Values

Normal values for ALT at 37°C is 6-30 U/L. The values are almost half when the reaction is carried out at 25°C.

Normal values (colorimetric methods)

serum ALT = 6-30 U/L
serum AST = 8-34 U/L

Clinical Relevance

High levels of serum AST activity are seen in the heart, liver, skeletal muscle and kidney tissues. Increased activity of AST in serum is observed in myocardial infarction after 20-36 hours of onset and hence used as a supporting evidence in the diagnosis of myocardial infarction. Values are usually less than 10 times the upper limit of normal (ULN). Increased activities are also observed in viral/toxic hepatitis, muscular dystrophy and in pulmonary embolism. ALT is distributed mainly in the liver and to a lesser extent in the kidney and muscles. Increased ALT activity is observed in hepatitis and cirrhosis. Values may be increased to more than 10–100 times ULN in hepatitis.

KIDNEY

Renal function tests are specialized tests and are advised when medical history, examination and routine tests like urine analysis are suggestive of some renal disease. Estimation of renal function s important in a number of clinical situations, including assessing renal damage and monitoring the progression of renal disease. Renal function should also be calculated if a potentially toxic drug is mainly cleared by renal excretion. The dose of the drug may need to be adjusted if renal function is abnormal.

Renal function tests may be grouped into (a) those, which assess the glomerular function, and (b) those, which study the tubular function.

Renal function tests are only for the analysis of the functional capacity of kidneys. Renal function tests do not give any information about the structural integrity or the structural pathology. For structural details renal imaging and biopsy has to be done.

The functional unit of the kidney is the nephron, which is composed of the glomerulus, proximal convoluted tubules (PCT), loop of Henle, distal convoluted tubules (DCT) and the collecting tubules. Quantitation of overall function of the kidneys is based on the assumption that all functioning nephrons are performing normally and that a decline in renal functions due to complete functional loss of nephrons rather than to compromised function of nephrons.

CREATININE

Estimation of blood creatinine and urea gives an approximate idea of renal impairment. However, in cases of moderate kidney damage, these levels might be within normal limits.

Estimation of Blood Creatinine (Jaffe's Test)—Principle

Creatinine is estimated by the Jaffe reaction. Creatinine reacts with alkaline picrate to give a colored complex. There are a number of other substances like glucose, uric acid, urea, protein, etc. that react with alkaline picrate. "True creatinine" value can be determined by getting rid of these nonspecific chromogens by the use of Lloyd's reagent which is hydrated aluminium silicate. Protein is precipitated with acid and the supernatant fluid is mixed with Lloyd's reagent which adsorbs creatinine in acid conditions. After centrifugation, the pellet is resuspended in alkaline picrate to elute the creatinine and the color reaction is developed.

Requirements

1. Sodium tungstate, 5% solution
2. Sulfuric acid solution, 2/3 N
3. Picric acid, 0.036 mol/L
4. NaOH solution, 0.75 N
5. Creatinine stock, 1 mg/ml in 0.1 N HCl. Dilute 1 : 25 before use (40 μg/ml)

Methodology

1. To 2 ml serum/plasma add 2.0 ml of water.
2. Add 2 ml of 5% sodium tungstate and 2.0 ml of 2/3 N H_2SO_4.
3. Mix and keep standing for 10 minutes.
4. Centrifuge and collect supernatant.
5. Take three tubes, T (Test), S (Standard) and B (Blank). Add 3 ml of supernatant (equivalent of 0.75 ml of original serum) to the test.
6. Then add 1 ml of picric acid and 1 ml of NaOH.
7. Develop the orange color for 20 minutes and record the absorbance at 520 nm.
8. For blank–Mix 4 ml distilled water, 2 ml tungstate and 2 ml sulfuric acid. Remove 3 ml from this mix and then add 1 ml each of picric acid and NaOH.
9. For standard–Mix 1 ml of working standard, 2 ml water, 2 ml tungstate, 2 ml sulfuric acid. Remove 3 ml from this mix and then add 1 ml each of picric acid and NaOH.
10. Read all tubes at 520 nm after 30 minutes.

Calculation

mg of creatinine/100 ml serum = [T/S] × [Conc. of stand/ml of serum taken] × 100

= [Reading of unknown/reading of standard] × [0.015/0.75] × 100

= [T/S] × 2

Normal Values

Adult males = 0.7–1.4 mg/dl
Adult females = 0.6 -1.3 mg/dl
Children = 0.4–1.2 mg/dl

Generally 'true' creatinine is 0.1 mg/dl lower than those given above.

Clinical Relevance

The kidney reserve is such that about 50% kidney function must be lost before the creatinine level in blood is raised. The creatinine concentration is hence a better indicator of renal function than blood urea or uric acid, because the creatinine levels are not affected by diet, exercise or hormones. A creatinine level of more than 1.5 mg/dl indicates impairment of renal function.

UREA

Urea contributes most of the body's non-protein nitrogen, accounting for about 45% of the total. It is the major end-product of protein catabolism in humans. It is synthesized in the liver, released into blood circulation and excreted by the kidneys. Measurement of urea in blood is a useful indicator of renal and hepatic integrity.

Estimation of Blood Urea (Diacetyl monoxime method)—Principle

Urea reacts directly with diacetyl monoxime under strong acidic conditions to give a yellow condensation product. The reaction is intensified by the presence of ferric ions and thiosemicarbazide. The intense red color formed is measured at 540 nm/yellow green filter.

Sample Collection

Serum is the specimen of choice. Store samples for no longer than 8 hours at room temperature (25-35°C) and 7 days at 2-8°C. For a longer duration, store in the freezer. If the samples show evidence of bacterial contamination, do not use these for urea estimation. Plasma could also be used for urea estimation.

Requirements

1. *Acid reagent*—Dissolve 1.0 g of ferric chloride hexahydrate in 30 ml of distilled water. Add 20 ml orthophosphoric acid and mix. Store in a brown bottle at room temperature (25-35°C). Stable for 6 months.
2. *Stock color reagent A*—Dissolve 2 g diacetyl monoxime in distilled water and make the volume up to 100 ml in a volumetric flask. Store in a brown bottle at room temperature (25-35°C). Stable for 6 months.
3. *Stock color reagent B*—Dissolve 0.5 g thiosemicarbazide in distilled water and make up to 100 ml in a volumetric flask. Store in a brown bottle at room temperature (25-35°C). Stable for 6 months.
4. *Mixed color reagent*—Mix 35 ml of stock color reagent A with 35 ml of stock color reagent B and make up to 500 ml with distilled water. Store in a brown bottle at room temperature (25-35°C). Stable for 6 months.
5. *Urea standard solution*—Weigh 1.0 g of analytical-grade urea and dissolve in 100 ml of benzoic acid (1g/dl). Use a 100 ml of volumetric flask for preparing this. Store at room temperature (25-35°C). Stable for 6 months. Dilute 1:20 before use.

Methodology

1. Pipette the following:

	S1	*S2*	*S3*	*Test*	*QC*
Distilled water (ml)	1.9	1.8	1.7	1.9	1.9
50 mg/dl urea (ml)	0.1	0.2	0.3	–	–
Test sample /QC (ml)	–	–	–	0.1	0.1

2. Pipette the following into another set of appropriately labeled tubes.

	Blank	*S1*	*S2*	*S3*	*Test*	*QC*
Color reagent (ml)	3.1	3.0	3.0	3.0	3.0	3.0
Respective diluted standard (ml)	–	0.1	0.1	0.1	–	–
Diluted test/QC (ml)	–	–	–	–	0.1	0.1

3. Mix all tubes well.
4. Keep them in a boiling water bath for 15 minutes.
5. Remove from water bath and cool the tubes for 5 minutes.
6. Set the spectrophotometer to zero with blank at 540 nm and measure the absorbance of the other tubes.

Calculation

Plot the absorbance values of standards against their respective concentrations. The measurable range with this graph is from 10 to 150 mg/dl. A calibration graph should be constructed whenever a new set of reagents is prepared. Plot absorbance values of test/QC on the calibration graph and read off the concentrations.

Normal Values

Serum/plasma urea .... 15–40 mg/dl

Clinical Relevance

Elevated serum urea levels may be due to prerenal, renal or post-renal etiology. Prerenal causes could be cardiac related or due to increased protein catabolism, and dehydration. Renal causes include glomerulonephritis, chronic nephritis, nephrotic syndrome and other kidney disease. Postrenal causes include obstruction of the urinary tract. Decreased serum urea levels could be due to pregnancy, intravenous infusion, low antidiuretic hormone secretion, low protein intake, severe liver diseases, inborn errors of urea cycle and SIADH (Syndrome of inappropriate ADH secretion).

GASTRIC JUICE

GASTRIC FUNCTION TESTS

The various motor and secretory activities of the stomach can be evaluated by a number of laboratory tests. These include:

a. Analysis of gastric residue, e.g. for blood, lactate, etc
b. Analysis of gastric secretions—before and after stimulation
c. Determination of intrinsic factor
d. Pepsinogen test
e. Tests for *Helicobacter pylori* (Endoscopy and serological test)

Some of these tests are more helpful in evaluating specific functions of the stomach for research purposes whereas others provide clinically important diagnostic data.

Measurements of gastric acidity can be used:

1. To detect the gross hypersecretion of acid in some cases of peptic ulcer and in Zollinger-Ellison syndrome (caused by gastrin producing tumor)
2. In the diagnosis of pernicious anemia
3. In gastric carcinoma—50% of patients show achlorhydria.

Preparation of the Patient

The patient should not eat, drink or smoke after dinner. The next morning, a nasogastric tube (Ryle's tube) is introduced in to the patient's stomach. The contents, aspirated and collected following 12 hours last is termed gastric residue". This can be analyzed for total acidity, occult blood; etc. After the stomach has been emptied, specimens are collected every 15 mins. Two specimens are collected. These are the secretions when the patient is at complete rest and not exposed to any visual auditory or olfactory stimulation. This 'basal secretion" is analyzed for free HCl and the result is reported in millimoles of free acid per hour (Basal acid output-BAO). Normal BAO is 1-2.5 ml/hour.

The parietal cell stimulant is then administered. The most commonly used stimulants are pentagastrin, histamine and histalog (given intramuscularly). Subsequent to the administration of the stimulant,

4 consecutive 15 ml samples are collected and they are labeled. These are analyzed for free HCl and the maximal acid output (MAO) is expressed in mmol/hour.

Estimation of Gastric Juice Features

Volume

In most normal cases after a night's fast only a small quantity (20 to 50 ml) of resting contents is obtained. Volumes above 100 to 120 ml may be considered abnormal. Increase in volume can be due to over secretion as in duodenal ulcer or Z.E. syndrome or due to delayed emptying due to pyloric obstruction.

Color

Fresh gastric juice is colorless or light yellow. Bright red, dark red or brown color can be due to the presence of blood. Blood may be present due to carcinoma of stomach, peptic ulcer or gastritis. Fresh blood may be due to accidental trauma from the gastric tube.

Miscellaneous Observations

Normal gastric secretion has an acidic odour. A disagreeable odour may be produced due to decayed food in gastric retention. Food particles in the gastric secretion indicate either a failure to fast or obstruction to gastric emptying. Organic acids if present are due to bacterial fermentation. Only pepsin is present in normal secretion. Trypsin can be present due to regurgitation.

pH

Normal pH of the gastric juice is 1.6-1.8.

Benzidine Test for Occult Blood

Requirements

1. Benzidine

Methodology

1. Mix 1 ml of benzidine and 0.5 ml of H_2O_2 with 1 ml of gastric juice.
2. Appearance of greenish blue color shows a positive test.

Part—V:

Future of Clinical Biochemistry

16

Future of Clinical Biochemistry

The clinical biochemistry is heading towards rapid automation and if most of the tests done today are heading for detection using simple and rapid kits or diagnostic equipments.

It began with need to have testing facilities as point-of-care testing (POCT) for immediate diagnostic assistance, rather than sending the samples all the way to clinical laboratories. POCT has also been called as 'near patient', 'beside' or 'extra-laboratory' testing. It can be considered as an evolutionary change in the mode of diagnostic testing wherein clinician can evaluate the patient and perform a test immediately to enhance his/her evaluation, then make a decision and take some form of action within the time frame of a single consultation. Throughout the world, the POCT is expanding at an amazing rate. In US alone it is growing at a rate of 12–15% and will see further increase only as POCT improves the therapeutic turn around time.

At one time, POCT was only used in hospital critical care testing areas (emergency and operating rooms). Now it is being used in clinics, physician's office and nursing homes. At the moment when the Buzz Words in laboratory practice include TQM (total quality management), GLP (Good laboratory practice) and SOP (standard operating procedures), the POCT systems provide a reliable solution. POCT devices can broadly be categorized into hand held and bench-top devices. The hand held devices are typified by the blood glucose test strips, urine strip tests and the more complex cassette type devices, which can be taken to the point where patient in under evaluation. The bench-top devices are often smaller version of systems originally designed for use in a laboratory, which includes systems meant for blood-gas analysis, electrolyte analysis, which have been recently extended to include devices for estimation of parathyroid hormone and cardiac markers.

In general, it is now possible to consider any analyte being measured using a POCT device, such is the level of innovation applied to this market. Thus it is now possible to use rapid immunoassay methods and molecular methods in addition to the electrochemical, colorimetric and enzymatic reactions. The advent of microfabrication of analytical devices and the consequent miniaturization of reaction cells with the faster reaction kinetics illustrate that the true needs of POCT–for the test result to be available within the same time frame that has been experienced with other diagnostic tools, e.g. the clinical thermometer, is soon to be realized.

The following points enlists the outcome of good POCT systems:

1. Reduced time of testing and decision–enhanced turnaround time
2. Reduced need of duplicate testing
3. Reduced utilization of drugs, clinical visits and a marked reduction in duration of stay
4. Increase in efficiency of health care facilities
5. More working man hours gained

So, in few words, the future of clinical biochemistry is of few minutes, small devices and of smaller labs, if any.

Part—VI:

Standards for the Tests

17

Standard Value Tables

BIOCHEMICAL FEATURES AND CONSTITUENTS IN BLOOD

Constituent/feature	*Concentration/normal value*
Acetoacetate, plasma	1 mg/dl
Albumin, serum	3.5–5.5 g/L
Aminotransferase	
Aspartate (SGOT)	0–35 U/L
Alanine (SGPT)	0–35 U/L
Ammonia, whole blood, venous	80–110 μg/dl
Amylase, serum	60–180 U/L
Ascorbic acid (Vitamin C)	0.4–1.0 mg/dl
β-hydroxybutyrate, plasma	< 3 mg/dl
Bilirubin, serum	0.3–1.0 mg/dl
Calciferol (Vitamin D)	16–65 pg/ml
Calcium, ionized	4.5–5.6 mg/dl
Calcium, plasma	9–10.5 mg/dl
Chlorides, serum	98-106 mEq/L
Cholesterol, total plasma	< 200 mg/dl
Cholesterol, LDL	< 130 mg/dl
Copper, serum	70–140 μg/dl
Creatinine, serum	1.5 mg/dl
Fatty acids, free plasma	18 mg/dl
Folic acid, red cells	150–450 ng/ml cells
Gastrin, serum	40–200 pg/ml
Globulins, serum	2.0–3.0 g/dl
Glucose	
Fasting, plasma	75–115 mg/dl
2 hours postprandial, plasma	< 140 mg/dl

Contd...

Contd...

Constituent/feature	*Concentration/normal value*
Hemoglobin, blood, sea level	
Male	14–16 g/dl
Female	12–16 g/dl
Iron, serum	50–150 μg/dl
Magnesium, serum	2–3 mg/dl
pH, blood	7.38–7.44
Phosphatase, acid, serum	0–5.5 U/L
Phosphatase, alkaline, serum	30–120 U/L
Phosphorus, inorganic, serum	3–4.5 mg/dl
Potassium, serum	3.5–5.0 mmol/L
Proteins, total serum	5.5–8.0 g/dl
Sodium, serum	136-145 mmol/L
Uric acid, serum	
Male	2.5–8.0 mg/dl
Female	1.5-6.0 mg/dl
Vitamin A, serum	20–100 μg/dl
Vitamin B_{12}, serum	200–600 pg/ml

CEREBROSPINAL FLUID

Feature	*Concentration/normal value*
Osmolarity	292–297 mmol/kg water
Electrolytes	
Sodium	137–145 mmol/L
Potassium	2.7–3.9 mmol/L
Calcium	1–1.5 mmol/L
Magnesium	1–1.2 mmol/L
Chloride	116–112 mmol/L
pH	7.31–7.34
Glucose	40–70 mg/dl
Lactate	10–20 mg/dl
Protein, total	20–50 mg/dl
Albumin	56-75%
Ammonia	25–80 μg/dl

Contd...

Contd...

Feature	*Concentration/normal value*
Creatinine	0.5-1.9 mg/dl
Pressure	50–180 mm H_2O
Volume	100–160 ml
Leukocytes, total	< 4 per ml

URINE

Feature	*Concentration/normal value*
Acidity, titratable	20–40 mmol/d
Ammonia	30–50 mmol/d
Calcium	200 mg/d
Copper	0–25 µg/d
Creatinine	
Male, Adult	< 50 mg/d
Female, Adult	< 100 mg/d
Glucose, true	50–300 mg/d
Protein	< 150 mg/d
Porphobilinogen	None
Potassium	25–100 mmol/d
Sodium	100–260 mmol/d
Urobilinogen	1–3.5 mg/d

AMNIOTIC FLUID

Feature	*Normal value*
Volume	800 ml (300-1400 ml) at term
Specific gravity	1.008
Color	Straw color
pH	72
Creatinine	2.2 mg/dl
Glucose	32 mg/dl
Urea	18 mg/dl

Contd...

Contd...

Feature	*Normal value*
Chloride	103 mg/dl
Sodium	126 mmol/L
Potassium	4.3 mmol/L
Protein, total	0.3 g/dl
Bilirubin, total	0.04 mg/dl
L/S	> 2
Uric acid	10.4 mg/dl

ADDITIONAL TABLES

RADIATION DERIVED UNITS

Quantity	*Old Unit*	*SI Unit*	*New Unit*	*Conversion*
Activity	curie (Ci)	disintegration per second	Becquerel	1 μCi = 37 GBq
Absorbed dose	rad	Joule per kilogram (J/kg)	gray (Gy)	1 Gy = 100 rad
Exposure	Roentgen(R)	Coulomb per kilogram (C/kg)	–	1 C/kg = 3798 R
Dose equivalent	rem	Joule per kilogram (J/kg)	Sievert (Sv)	1 Sv = 100 rem

UNITS USED IN THE BOOK

Symbol	*Representation of*	*Standard denotion*	*Derivation wrt normal value*
sec	Time	Hour	3600 sec = 1 hour
min			60 min = 1 hour
h			Standard value
d			24 hour = 1 day
ml	Volume	Milliliter	Standard value
dl			10 ml = 1 dl
L			1000 ml = 1 L
pg	Weight	Gram	1 gm = 10^{12} pg
ng			1 gm = 10^{9} ng
μg			1 gm = 10^{6} mg
mg			1 gm = 10^{3} mg
g			Standard value
kg			1000 gm = 1 kg
M, mmol	Concentration	—	Gm. Mol. wt. of compound/L.

INDEX